FUNCTIONAL COMPUTED TOMOGRAPHY

Edited by

Kenneth Miles

Southern X-ray Clinics, Wesley Hospital, Chasely Street, Brisbane 4066, Australia

Peter Dawson

Department of Diagnostic Radiology, Hammersmith Hospital, Du Cane Road, London W12 0NN, UK

Martin Blomley

Department of Diagnostic Radiology, Hammersmith Hospital, Du Cane Road, London W12 0NN, UK

ISIS MEDICAL MEDIA

Oxford

To Anne

First published 1997

British Library Cataloguing in Publication Data. A catalogue record for this title is available from the British Library

ISBN 1 899066 39 X

Miles, K (Kenneth)
Functional computed tomography
Kenneth Miles, Peter Dawson and Martin Blomley

Always refer to the manufacturer's Prescribing Information before prescribing drugs cited in this book.

Typeset by
EXPO Holdings Sdn Bhd., Malaysia

Printed in Hong Kong

Distributed in the USA by
Mosby-Year Book, Inc.
11830 Westline Industrial Drive
St Louis, MO63146, USA

Distributed in the rest of the world by
Oxford University Press
Saxon Way West, Corby,
Northants NN18 9ES, UK

CONTENTS

PREFACE

Until recently, the main thrust within radiology has been towards the assessment of disease through demonstrating changes in structure. The body of knowledge within pathology has largely provided the basis of this approach. New developments in imaging, particularly the use of computers in image acquisition and processing, have been associated with the emergence of approaches aimed at assessing disease through changes in organ function.

This new approach has come at a time when genetics has emerged as a major topic within medicine. Rather than being merely coincidental, genetics and functional imaging are connected by the fact that genes are primarily expressed as a change in tissue function, for instance as a particular surface receptor or by the release of angiogenetic factors.

This new functional approach should not be competitive with structural imaging but complementary. This is exemplified by the use of computed tomography (CT) to image organ function thereby combining physiological information with the already proven benefits of structural CT. At a time of increasing cost restraint within healthcare, functional CT also benefits from fulfilling both approaches within one examination and without the need of additional equipment.

This book aims to describe the current status of functional imaging with CT. The scientific basis of the methodology is described in detail and a practical approach to acquiring and processing the image data is given. The results obtained from studying normal organs are presented and subsequently compared to those derived from patients in a clinical setting. Although much of the content is currently within the research domain, the recent rapid growth in the number of slip-ring CT systems means that there is great potential to bring the benefits of these functional CT techniques to a large number of patients within the clinical arena.

Kenneth Miles
Peter Dawson
Martin Blomley

Chapter 1
INTRODUCTION TO FUNCTIONAL COMPUTED TOMOGRAPHY

K. Miles and P. Dawson

HISTORICAL PERSPECTIVE

Within a very short space of time following their discovery by Röntgen in 1895, it was widely realized that X-rays could be used to visualize the internal anatomy of the human body. As diagnostic radiology has developed, this emphasis on the demonstration of disease through changes in morphology has remained. Although the development of X-ray contrast media did allow some qualitative judgements about function to be made during radiological examinations, such as intravenous urography or angiography, quantitative measurements have not been practicable due to the inconvenience and unreliability of film densitometric analysis.

Historically, imaging of changes in the *function* of organs has been achieved primarily by the determination of the distribution of radioactive substances within the body and this dichotomy of 'radiology for structure and nuclear medicine for function' has persisted until quite recently. Although exhibiting poor spatial resolution, nuclear medicine techniques are very well suited to functional imaging. The detectors are extremely sensitive and can detect very small quantities of administered radiopharmaceuticals. This means that the mass of chemical administered is so small that it does not itself affect the function of the organ system under study — the basis and *sine qua non* of the 'tracer' concept. A further strength is the ability to quantify the amount of tracer by simply counting the number of photons detected. A number of mathematical analyses have been developed to allow more precise physiological data to be extracted, particularly from temporal changes in radioisotope concentrations within organs and the blood. With the introduction of gamma cameras linked to computers, such data processing advanced further with computer generation of datasets from regions of interest and, ultimately, from individual pixels. The use of individual pixel datasets led ultimately to the production of parametric images where the value attributed to a pixel is a physiological measure derived by calculation using data from that pixel position for each image of a sequence. Today, such techniques of analysis are used routinely, for instance in positron emission tomography.

The introduction of small computers also had a profound impact upon diagnostic radiology by leading to the development of new imaging technologies that used computers either to control the imaging apparatus or, more importantly, to acquire primary data in digital format. This included the development of X-ray computed tomography (CT) which brilliantly synthesized established technologies by harnessing the computer to the problem of image-slice reconstruction. However, when Sir Godfrey Hounsfield and co-workers first described CT in 1973, it was, once again, its exceptional ability to demonstrate internal *anatomy*, particularly of the brain, that caught the attention of radiologists. In fact, the potential value of quantitative measurements of X-ray attenuation (CTW^{as}), was an early realization and it was hoped that such measurements would allow differentiation of different pathologies. However, this proved to be limited in practice to the determination of the fat or calcium content of tissues or to the demonstration of fluid-filled cysts. Such hopes were raised again when intravascular contrast agents were used in CT. Some tissues were found to enhance more or less than others but the true potential for tissue characterization remained limited.

Despite the parallel developments occurring in nuclear medicine, the potential for CT to provide quantitative assessments of organ function remained unrealized until 1980 when Axel [1] proposed a method for determination of cerebral blood flow by analysis of data from a rapid sequence of CT images performed without table movement. The delay of seven years since the introduction of CT was largely a result of the inability of early CT systems to acquire rapid series of image datasets due to the translocate/rotate mode of action of the first-generation CT equipment. The rotate-only action of second-generation systems and improvements in X-ray tube design enabled the development of 'dynamic CT'. Rapid sequences could now be performed with or without table movement and became known, respectively, as 'incremental' and 'single-location' sequences. The incremental sequences gained in popularity as they enabled the whole of an organ to be visualized during the period of maximal enhancement following intravenous administration of contrast media. Once again, the radiologist with a traditional interest in form rather than function, was the driving force.

With a few notable exceptions, such as the demonstration of dissection of the thoracic aorta, the application of single-location sequences remained more limited. Many reports comprised empirical studies of tissue time–density measurements following contrast media in an attempt to achieve tissue characterization. Although successful in some circumstances, such as in the diagnosis of cavernous haemangioma of the liver, the potential for tissue characterization appeared limited. In retrospect, this is perhaps not surprising as such analysis did not take variations in the vascular input into account. This is despite the fact that experience from nuclear medicine had shown the importance of the 'input function' in determining temporal changes in tissue concentrations of tracers. The same problem exists today with much of the current gadolinium-enhanced dynamic magnetic resonance research, though here there is at least the excuse that an input function depending only on gadolinium concentration is genuinely difficult to obtain, since signal is influenced by flow itself.

A few workers did undertake a more basic physiological approach. The first report on functional CT was published, as indicated earlier, in 1980 [1] when Axel described a method for determination of cerebral perfusion from dynamic CT data. A year later, Ishikawa *et al.* reported that renal function could be estimated by determining the time at which renal cortical and medullary time–density curves crossed [2]. Jansen *et al.* adapted the nuclear medicine concept of perfusion index by comparing the slopes of renal cortical and aortic time–density curves in the evaluation of renal transplants [3]. Some researchers used other nuclear medicine data-processing techniques to measure physiological processes, such as tissue perfusion, in absolute units. Herfkens *et al.* used the Stewart–Hamilton approach to measure cardiac output with CT [4] and determined the mean transit time (MTT) of tissues through deconvolution of dynamic CT data. On the technological side, the development of electron beam ultrafast CT systems with no moving parts enabled very rapid dataset acquisitions and made possible the measurement of cardiac perfusion [5].

An alternative approach to obtaining functional information from CT has been the use of stable xenon as a contrast medium. Cerebral perfusion can be determined from the rate of wash-in (and sometimes wash-out) of xenon in different brain regions. The amount of brain enhancement, and hence the signal-to-noise ratio, is limited by the administered concentration of xenon gas. At a concentration of 80%, xenon is a potent anaesthetic and even concentrations of 50–60% may cause sedation, bronchospasm or respiratory depression; 33% xenon (with 67% oxygen) is tolerated by 90% of patients and yet transient sensory disturbances or occasionally respiratory depression occur. Such effects increase the probability of artefacts due to movement of the patient. Blood pressure, arterial oxygen saturation, end tidal CO_2 concentration and respiratory rate must also be monitored continuously during the study. Xenon also causes flow activation within the brain. These problems and the need for specialized equipment have meant that application of the technique has remained limited.

OVERVIEW OF FUNCTIONAL IMAGING

More recently, there has been a general shift in emphasis within radiology away from purely anatomical imaging towards a combined structural–functional approach. This has resulted from the development of many new imaging techniques that use digital information in the image acquisition process; these include not just CT, but also magnetic resonance imaging (MRI), ultrasound and digital angiography. The approach also embraces new nuclear medicine technologies and radiotracers which provide functional information that can be co-registered with anatomical images from other modalities using computers. The range of functions is broad and is summarized in Figure 1.1.

Functional imaging techniques that exploit modalities more conventionally used for anatomical imaging include MRI measurements of vessel flow, tissue

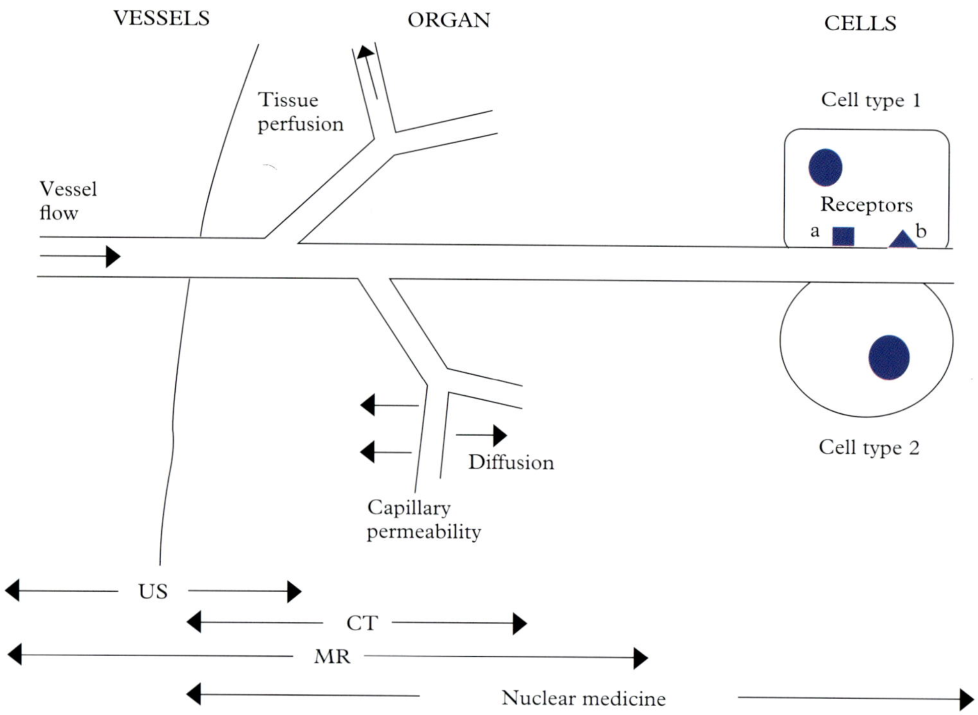

Figure 1.1
Relationship between functional imaging techniques and organ structure. US = ultrasound; CT = computed tomography; MR = magnetic resonance.

perfusion and diffusion, Doppler ultrasound measurements of blood velocity and, with the use of ultrasonic contrast media, tissue perfusion determination, and assessment of vessel flow and renal function by digital angiography.

However, nuclear medicine currently remains the only technique that can evaluate detailed cellular function. The functional specificity of different tracers enables different cell types, or even different functions (e.g. receptors) within one cell type, to be distinguished. Thus nuclear medicine techniques have high 'functional resolution', evaluating microscopic cellular elements that are too small to be resolved using anatomical imaging techniques such as CT or MRI. Unfortunately, nuclear medicine images are of relatively poor spatial resolution and therefore any abnormalities of cellular function cannot be accurately located. Nuclear medicine images can be co-registered with anatomical images from other modalities with some improvement in spatial localization but problems with misregistration remain.

But why image function at all? The development of functional imaging within radiology is akin to the introduction of cytohistochemical techniques to pathology. Through identification of certain chemical or immunological features of cells, such histological techniques have allowed improved accuracy of diagnosis and reclassification of diseases with closer correlation to prognosis and treatment. Similar benefits can be anticipated as a result of the improved tissue characterization and greater detail of information about disease processes that is provided by functional imaging but with the advantage that these benefits can be achieved non-invasively in the living patient rather than from a pathological specimen obtained at biopsy, surgery or postmortem.

Thus, there are many benefits to be anticipated from the development of functional imaging. Firstly, disease detection may be improved as functional changes often occur in pathological processes before any structural change is readily apparent. Secondly, the tissue characterization afforded by functional imaging may enable identification of pathologies that are indistinguishable on morphological criteria. In some cases, this may obviate biopsy. Similarly, functional imaging may identify subgroups of patients with a particular disease between which there may be a difference in prognosis or in whom specific treatments are more or less likely to be of benefit. This may allow potentially harmful treatment regimes to be reserved for patients most likely to benefit whilst enabling treatments with unpleasant side effects to be avoided when no benefit is to be expected, for instance, with certain cancer chemotherapy regimes. Thirdly, functional imaging may demonstrate response to treatments before any improvement can be detected on morphological grounds. Such improvements in diagnostic accuracy should lead to the instigation of more appropriate management and improved outcomes.

CT AS A TECHNIQUE FOR FUNCTIONAL IMAGING

This book describes CT techniques that allow measurement of physiological processes through determination of the temporal changes in X-ray attenuation occurring after intravenous administration of conventional contrast media. The imaging protocols are developments of dynamic CT techniques and involve repeated data acquisitions without table movement. The data processing methods are largely adaptations of nuclear medicine methodology allowing measurement of tissue perfusion, blood volume, renal function and capillary permeability. Functional CT is not only a valuable research tool but a number of clinical applications are also emerging.

CT is well suited to functional imaging. Unlike the situation with MRI and ultrasound contrast media, there is a linear relationship between the concentration of iodinated contrast media and background-subtracted CT measurements of attenuation and therefore time–density data, readily amenable to data-processing techniques used in nuclear medicine, are obtainable. Reference data from the vascular system can be readily obtained without arterial sampling by including a suitable blood vessel within the area of study. The spatial resolution is good, enabling structural and functional information to be combined in the one study whilst avoiding the misregistration errors associated with multimodality image fusion. The techniques use conventional contrast media and require no special equipment (beyond a personal computer). Although primarily chosen for performing spiral or helical techniques, the introduction and widespread installation of slip-ring CT systems has meant that functional CT is now a technique available to many radiology departments throughout the world.

REFERENCES

1. Axel, L. (1980) Cerebral blood flow determination by rapid-sequence computed tomography; theoretical analysis. *Radiology*, **137**, 679–686.
2. Ishikawa, I., Onouchi, Z., Saito, Y. *et al.* (1981) Renal cortex visualisation and analysis of dynamic CT curves of the kidney. *Journal of Computer Assisted Tomography*, **5**, 695–701.
3. Jansen, V.O., Gmelin, E., Burmester, E. *et al.* (1989) Analyse von dynamischen CT-kurven bei nierentransplantaten mit abstossungsreaktion und cyclosporin-A-intoxikation. Röentgen Fortschrift, **151**, 473–476.
4. Herfkens, R.J., Axel, L., Lipton, M.J. *et al.* (1982) Measurement of cardiac output by computed transmission tomography. *Invest Radiol*, **17**, 550–553.
5. Wolfkiel, C.J., Ferguson, J.L., Chomka, E.V. *et al.* (1987) Measurement of myocardial blood flow by ultrafast computed tomography. *Circulation*, **761**, 1262–1273.

Chapter 2

PROCESSING CT DATA FOR FUNCTIONAL STUDIES

M. Hayball

INTRODUCTION

This chapter discusses the problems associated with access to X-ray computed tomography (CT) images and postprocessing of the data to produce functional information from dynamic, single-location, contrast-enhanced image sets. Although a few CT consoles have the facilities for some functional analyses, this is rarely sufficient and access to an external workstation will be required to implement the techniques described here.

EVALUATION OF CT SYSTEMS FOR FUNCTIONAL IMAGING

Requirements for CT systems differ depending on the range of functional processing required. First-pass studies — those which assume the administered contrast medium is retained in the vessels during the examination — require a system with a fast imaging time of approximately 1 s per slice, whereas longer studies such as the Patlak permeability-measurement protocol require images taken at 15–20 s intervals and place lower demands on the CT system. The production of functional images requires good reproducibility and low noise within the data. If only region of interest (ROI) analysis is required, the reproducibility and noise are unlikely to cause problems in a clinically acceptable CT system.

Duration and repetition speed

Most first-pass functional imaging techniques require a system capable of acquiring a single location dynamic dataset of 10–15 images over a period of 40–60 s. Figures 2.1 and 2.2 show the effect of acquisition time and interscan delay on the time–density curves for a typical arterial enhancement. It can be seen that an interscan delay of 3 s and scan duration of 1 s gives an adequate estimate of the true time–density curve for first-pass studies. An increase of the scan duration to 2 s is likely to reduce the measured enhancement due to an averaging effect.

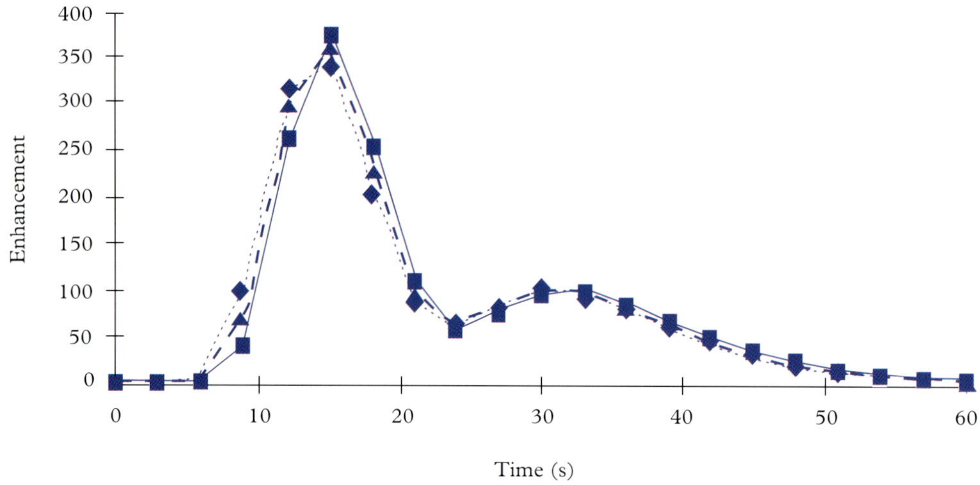

Figure 2.1
The effect of scan duration on the estimated enhancement within a vessel. Data points are generated from an idealized time–density curve based on real data. Calculated data points as would be generated by the given acquisition parameters are:
—■— = delay 3 s, duration 0 s;
– –▲– – = delay 3 s, duration 1 s;
····◆···· = delay 3 s, duration 2 s.

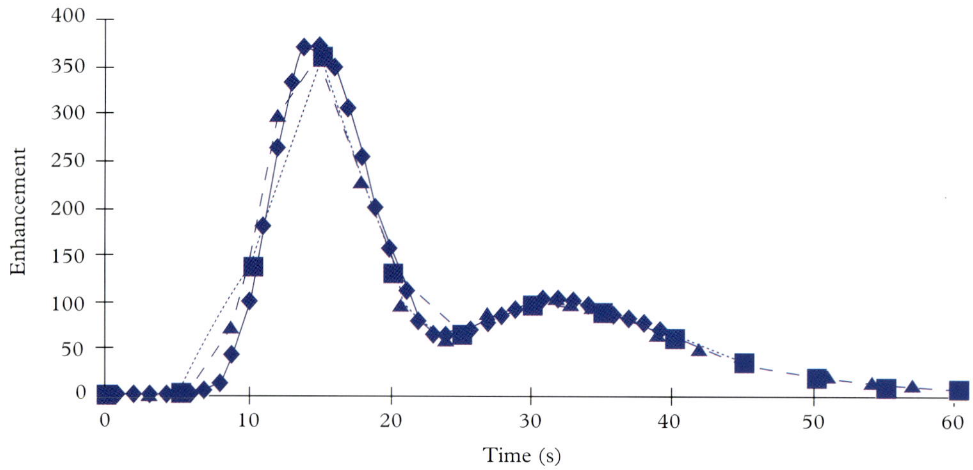

Figure 2.2
The effect of interscan delay on the estimated enhancement within a vessel. Data points are generated from an idealized time–density curve based on real data. Calculated data points as would be generated by the given acquisition parameters are:
—◆— = delay 1 s, duration 0 s;
– –▲– – = delay 3 s, duration 1 s;
····■···· = delay 5 s, duration 1 s.

Increase of the interscan delay may lead to the peak enhancement being missed and may reduce the accuracy of the gradient measurement.

Noise

Noise as seen in time–density curves has two main causes. The first is related to the reproducibility; the second is related to patient movement.

If a series of identical measurements are made, there will be some fluctuation of the CT number determined. This reproducibility error depends on a number of factors. The mAs value for the image will affect the number of photons detected — the number of photons should be proportional to the mAs for an image. Noise due to quantization error should thus be reduced with the square root of the mAs value. The kV setting for the image will affect the X-ray attenuation and detector efficiency and hence may change the quantization error, though this relationship is not a simple one.

The reconstruction algorithm plays an important part in the reproducibility. Soft-tissue reconstruction algorithms tend to have a smoothing effect on the image, reducing the noise, whereas high-resolution algorithms tend to increase noise. Any artefact on the images will interfere with the tissue-perfusion calculation by artificially changing the CT enhancement. Most commonly, these are produced by beam hardening around dense objects, poor detector calibration or movement of the patient. Artefacts can be reduced by reducing the slice thickness at the expense of a decrease in the signal-to-noise ratio. It is expected of a modern machine that it will regularly recalibrate all its detectors and hence image uniformity should never be a problem.

An important potential reproducibility error arises when partial reconstruction is used to reduce the scan duration — for example, a 270° rotation on a machine with a 2 s rotation time can give a 1.5 s scan duration. If the partial reconstruction does not start at the same point for each slice, the differences in the raw data used by the reconstruction algorithm can lead to slight changes in the CT numbers calculated.

If an object being imaged is not completely uniform, any slight movement will mean that repeated measurements will vary depending on the magnitude of the movement and variation of the object density. The motion noise will vary depending on the organ being viewed and the size of the voxel or region of interest.

The noise due to the CT machine can be estimated by taking images of a water phantom under the same conditions as the dynamic series. The following sample assessment was performed on the Somaton Plus (Siemens, Ehrlangen, Germany) at Addenbrooke's Hospital.

1. Three scans were performed for the standard reconstruction algorithm and the soft-tissue reconstruction algorithm. The images produced were transferred to the workstation and compressed to a 256 × 256 matrix. A region 40 pixels square was created and the variation of values within this region was analysed. The temporal variation of a single voxel was found to be very similar to the spatial variation within a single slice. The amplitude of noise (calculated as the standard deviation of voxel values) for the standard reconstruction algorithm was found to be 3.2 Hounsfield units (HU). That for the soft-tissue reconstruction algorithm was found to be 2.7 HU.
2. A similar process was performed on a 20 pixel square region positioned in liver tissue for three consecutive scans taken before contrast reached the tissue and using the standard soft-tissue algorithm. This gives an indication of the typical variation in measurements above which the change in contrast must be measured. The spatial variation within a scan gave a standard deviation of 4.4 HU and the temporal variation of a voxel, a standard deviation of 3.9 HU. The difference between these figures can be explained by the expected

physiological variation of density in the liver. This will be seen as variation of voxel value with position but will not be seen as a variation with time unless there is patient movement. The increase in variation compared with the water phantom is probably due to increased attenuation.

The effect of noise on measurements and functional images is treated later in this chapter.

ACCESS TO IMAGE DATA

Some CT systems provide facilities for generation of time–density curves from regions of interest. Processing of these curves is usually limited but the enhancement values can usually be printed in table form. These data can be entered manually into a spreadsheet for processing. For more interactive processing, a means for transfer to an independent workstation will usually be required. Most CT systems now come with the facilities to transfer images to external workstations although some older systems use proprietary data formats where image transfer is more problematic.

A collection of up-to-date information on image-storage formats and techniques for transfer of image data from a wide range of scanners is available in the excellent 'frequently asked questions' (FAQ) list maintained by David Clunie. The FAQ is posted to the Usenet conference *alt.image.medical* and available from the web site at *http://www.rahul.net/dclunie/html/*.

On-line and archive storage of reconstructed images is almost always in a proprietary data format. Archive storage is usually on magneto-optical disk with optional storage on tape. Although manufacturers may release the data formats, it is not usually a simple matter to read the data directly from the archive media and a network link is preferable.

Digital imaging and communications in medicine

Almost all new CT equipment provides Digital Imaging and Communications in Medicine (DICOM) connectivity. The DICOM 3.0 standards have grown from the American College of Radiologists/National Equipment Manufacturers Association (ACR/NEMA) standards for image transfer. In its initial form, it defined a means for equipment and workstations from different manufacturers to negotiate communication and transfer images over a network. It should be noted that, at present, it does not define a storage format. A number of low-cost PC-based viewing stations are now available which will accept the transfer of images using the DICOM protocol. Most of these provide an option to store the data on disk in a DICOM-like format but often the classification of images by patient, study, etc. may be stored in a proprietary database. DICOM connectivity is a complex subject — the FAQ and the DICOM resources web

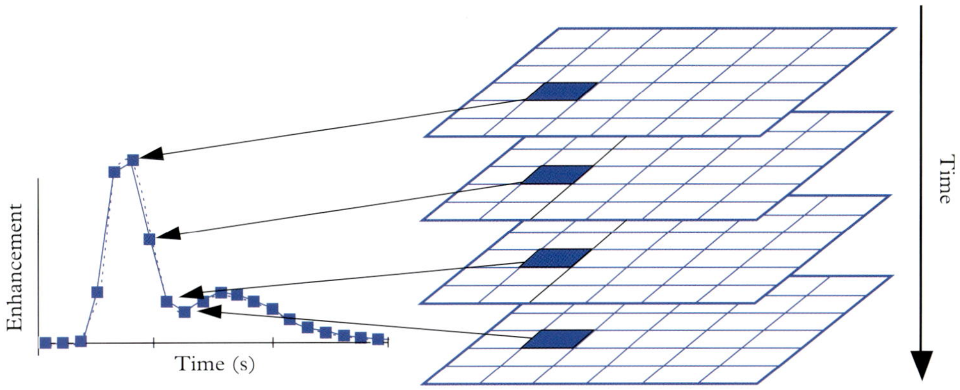

Figure 2.3 Creation of a time–density curve from a sequence of images. Each voxel contributes to a single point on the time–density curve.

site at *http://www.merge.com/subpage/DICOM.html* are good sources of information.

DERIVATION OF TIME–DENSITY CURVES

Time–density (time–attenuation) curves are generated by measuring the average CT number in a voxel or region of interest at a number of time points following the administration of a bolus of iodinated contrast. The presence of iodinated contrast increases the density of tissue in a voxel by an amount proportional to its concentration. The CT number (given in HU) is proportional to density over a limited range and for the purposes of this technique any non-linearity in the conversion of CT number to density is unlikely to be significant. The constant of proportionality is not required for the techniques described here. By subtracting the value of the first, precontrast slice (the reference slice) from all the subsequent points, the time–density curve can be adjusted to show only the enhancement due to the presence of contrast and any reproducibility or movement-induced errors. The time values for the time–density curve are determined from the delay of subsequent slices after the reference slice. Figure 2.3 illustrates the generation of a time–density curve from voxels within an image.

When generating a time–density curve from a ROI, the contribution of any variation generated by the system is reduced as the square root of the number of voxels in the region and, hence, unless very small regions are used, it is unlikely to be necessary to use any smoothing on the data. A more common problem, however, is the inclusion of voxels containing larger vessels, the presence of which may invalidate an algorithm which assumes that the region contains only tissue. This is a particular problem in the brain where it is difficult to position a ROI without including any significant vessels. Similarly, if a region contains bone or air, this may result in an increased sensitivity to movement. The solution to

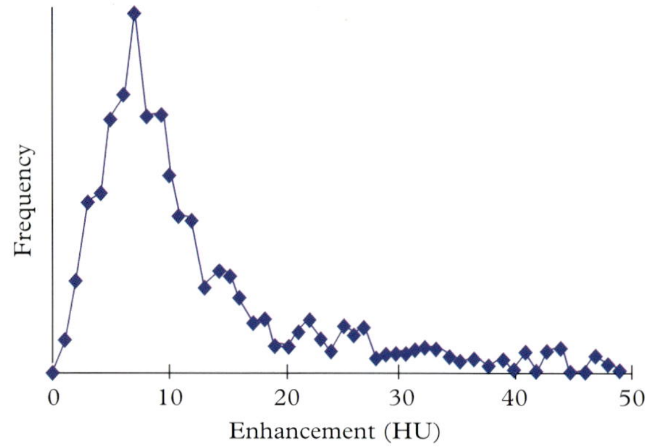

Figure 2.4
A histogram of maximum enhancement values within the region shown in Figure 2.5(a). This can be used to determine the most suitable threshold values for the elimination of vessels.

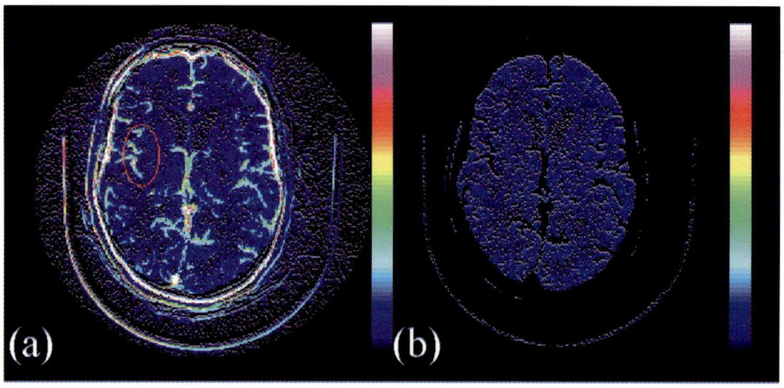

Figure 2.5
Maximum enhancement image derived from images in Figure 2.7. Colour scale shows range of enhancement 0 to 100 HU. (a) The enhancement derived without time–density curve filtering. (b) The enhancement with time–density curve filtering set to exclude vessels (initial CT number –5 to 400 HU, enhancement range –5 to 20 HU).

this problem is to exclude voxels from the region if they fail certain criteria. Two sets of thresholds can be applied. The first is applied only to the first image of the sequence and is set to exclude bone and air. A range of 0 to 100 HU is suitable. The second threshold is applied to the subsequent points after subtraction of the reference image. If vessels are to be included, this should be set above the maximum enhancement expected: a range of –10 to 400 HU is usually adequate as it allows for small errors in the measurement of the reference image and the administered contrast will rarely exceed an enhancement of 350 HU. If vessels are to be excluded, then the value depends on the tissue to be analysed. For example, a range of –5 to 20 HU in the brain and –10 to 100 HU in the abdomen improves image quality.

A suitable threshold can be selected using a histogram of enhancement values. Figure 2.4 shows a histogram generated from a region within the brain containing both tissue and vessel. Figures 2.5 and 2.6 show images derived, with and without this threshold applied, from the brain-perfusion dataset shown in Figure 2.7. Figure 2.8 shows a similar treatment for a liver-perfusion dataset.

Where the time–density curve is to be derived from a voxel within an image, the errors due to reproducibility and movement become more significant and it is often necessary to smooth the data before deriving functional information. This

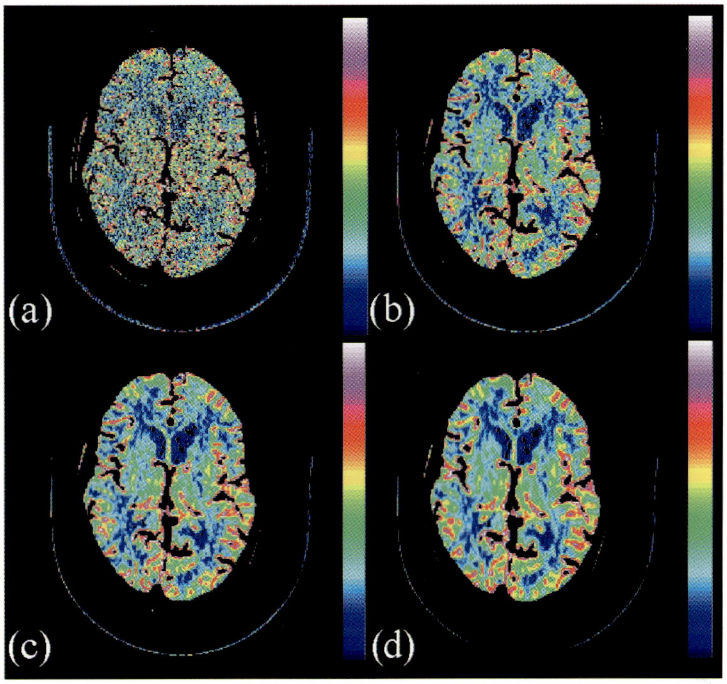

Figure 2.6
Maximum enhancement image derived from images in Figure 2.7 with threshold filtering applied. Colour scale shows range of enhancement 0 to 20 HU. Image (a) shows image derived with no spatial smoothing applied. Images (b), (c) and (d) employ smoothing kernels of degree 1, 2 and 3, respectively.

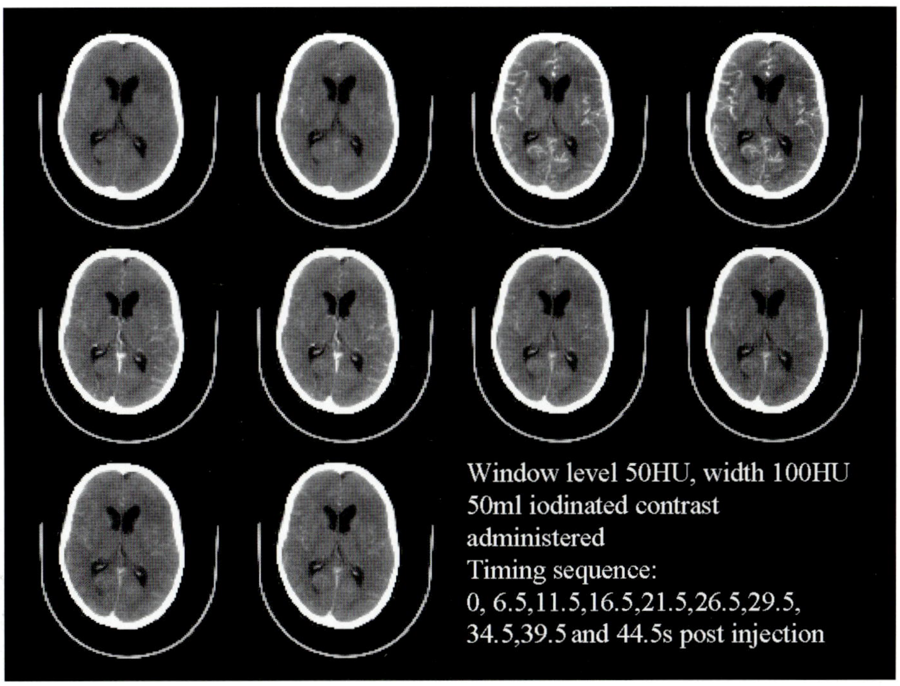

Figure 2.7
Sequence of images for investigation of brain perfusion.

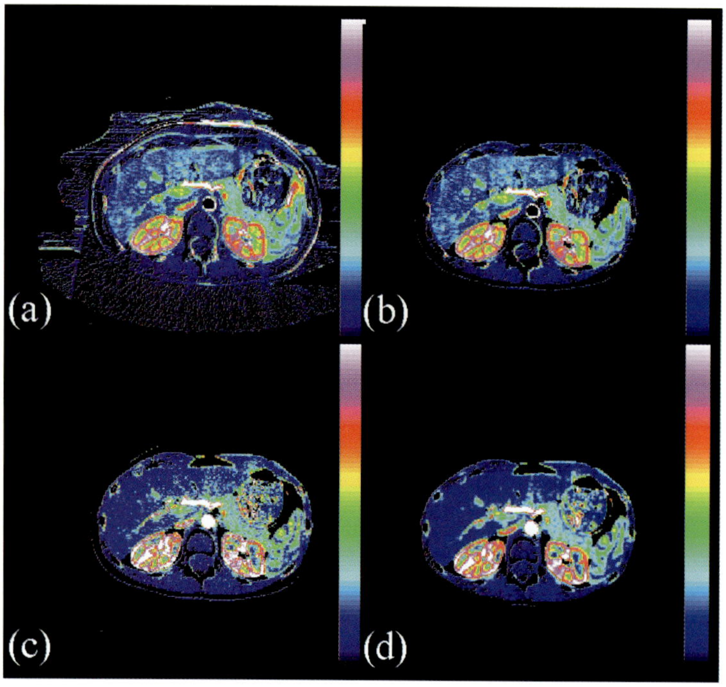

Figure 2.8
Enhancement and perfusion images derived from abdomen images. Colour scale shows range of enhancement of 0 to 200 HU for images (a) and (b) and range of perfusion of 0 to 5.0 ml/min/ml for images (c) and (d). Image (a) shows image derived with no spatial smoothing applied and no time–density curve filtering. Images (b), (c) and (d) have time–density curve filtering (initial CT number −100 to 1000 HU, enhancement range −100 to 1000 HU) to remove artefact. Image (d) employs a smoothing kernel of degree 1.

can be achieved by applying a binomial smoothing kernel to the raw data in each slice. The smoothing kernels used are as follows:

$$\overline{K} = \frac{1}{16}\begin{pmatrix} 1 & 2 & 1 \\ 2 & 4 & 2 \\ 1 & 2 & 1 \end{pmatrix} \text{for smoothing of degree 1,}$$

$$\overline{K} = \frac{1}{256}\begin{pmatrix} 1 & 4 & 6 & 4 & 1 \\ 4 & 16 & 24 & 16 & 4 \\ 6 & 24 & 36 & 24 & 6 \\ 4 & 16 & 24 & 16 & 4 \\ 1 & 4 & 6 & 4 & 1 \end{pmatrix} \text{for degree 2.}$$

The smoothed value for point P_{ij} is given by:

$$S_{i,j} = \sum_{k=0}^{2n+1} \sum_{l=0}^{2n+1} \overline{K}P_{\mathrm{i}+k-n,j+l-n} \text{ where } n \text{ is the degree of smoothing.}$$

The degree of smoothing required to produce an acceptable functional image depends on the algorithm and voxel size and can be quite subjective. Abdominal images using a 256 voxel square matrix will usually benefit from smoothing with $n = 1$, brain images often require smoothing of $n = 3$ to 4. Figures 2.6, 2.8 and 2.9 show the effect of smoothing on some sample images.

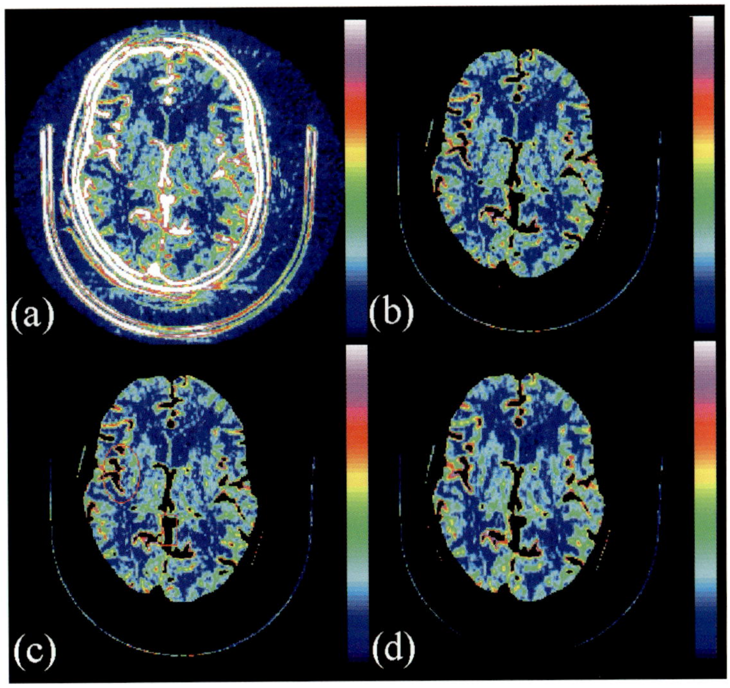

Figure 2.9
Perfusion images derived from images in Figure 2.7. Colour scale shows range of perfusion of 0 to 2.0 ml/min/ml. Image (a) shows an image derived with no spatial smoothing applied and no threshold filter. Images (b), (c) and (d) employ smoothing kernels of degree 1, 2 and 3, respectively.

When a large number of noisy images are acquired, as is the case in some nuclear scintigraphy studies or using electron-beam CT, temporal smoothing may be desirable. In standard X-ray CT acquisitions, however, this should not be required.

DERIVATION OF FUNCTION INFORMATION FROM A TIME–DENSITY CURVE

Having derived the time–density curve for a region or voxel, interpolation is usually required to produce a continuous curve from which parametric information can be derived. Simple linear interpolation can be used but this can lead to underestimation of the maxima and measurement of time to maximum is accurate only to the nearest point on the curve. Cubic interpolation produces a smoothly varying curve which allows more accurate estimation of these parameters. Figure 2.10 compares these two techniques and the Appendix (page 25) gives details of the interpolation algorithms.

An alternative to interpolation is the use of a mathematical model for the time–density curve. The gamma variate is often used to describe the shape of a bolus in nuclear medicine. A selection of gamma-variate curves is shown in Figure 2.11. Various methods exist for the determination of the gamma-variate curve which best matches the time–density curve. Fitting the gamma-variate

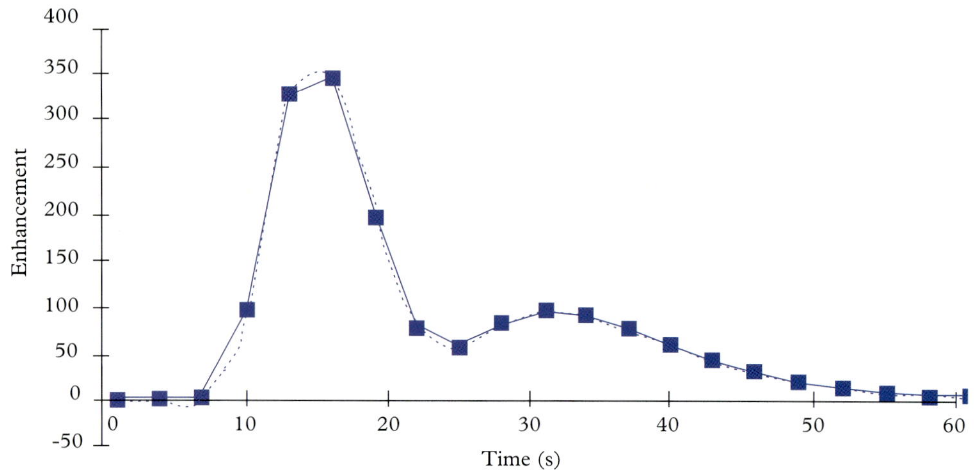

Figure 2.10
The effect of the interpolation on the estimation of a time–density curve. ——■—— = linear interpolation; ·········· = cubic spline

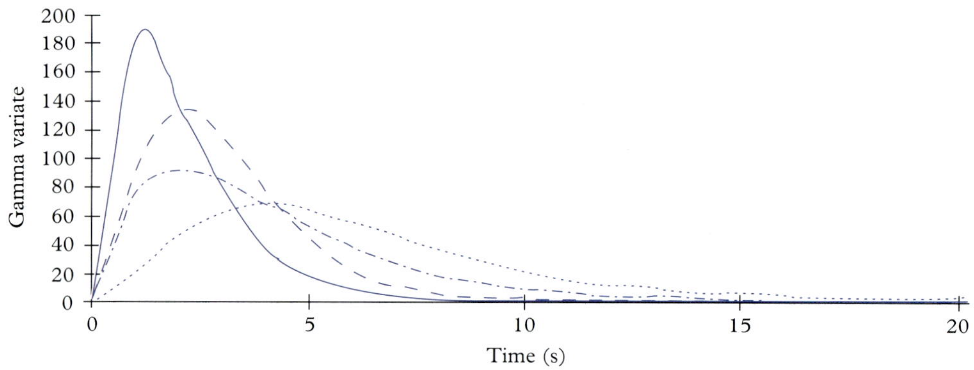

Figure 2.11
A selection of gamma-variate curves, having parameters $\alpha = 1$, $\beta = 1$; $\alpha = 2$, $\beta = 1$; $\alpha = 1$, $\beta = 2$; $\alpha = 2$, $\beta = 2$. t_a is 0 in each case and k is chosen such that the area under each curve is the same. ———— = curve 1; – – – – = curve 2; –·–·–·– = curve 3; ·········· = curve 4.

curve to the data is computationally intensive and is not suitable for tissues such as the liver which have both arterial and portal blood supply or when recirculation occurs before the enhancement has reduced significantly from the initial bolus. Both of these cases require the summation of two or more gamma-variate curves — a process which is difficult to automate. The process has, however, been successfully implemented for ROI studies in the heart [1,2]. Once the gamma-variate curve fitting has been performed, curve parameters such as maximum enhancement and time to maximum can be derived directly from the gamma variate. The Appendix gives details of one such method and some characteristics of the curve.

Examples of algorithms

The following examples illustrate a number of parameters which can be derived from the image and algorithms required. It is assumed in each case that the time–density curve represents the increase above that of the reference image of the CT number for each scan in a time sequence.

Maximum enhancement and time to maximum

The maximum enhancement and time to maximum values are the easiest parameters to determine and though they are not directly related to any physiological function, they can be useful indicators of relative perfusion and transit time. A maximum enhancement image is very useful when searching for a suitable vessel to use as an input to one of the functional algorithms below. If simple linear interpolation is used, then the maximum enhancement value is simply the maximum value within the time–density curve and the time to maximum, the scan delay for that slice. This is adequate for many maximum enhancement calculations but the time resolution is limited to the interscan delay (typically 3 s) and this is rarely accurate enough. Cubic interpolation is advised for the measurement of time to peak. The calculations required for cubic interpolation can be reduced by first finding the maximum using linear interpolation and then applying cubic interpolation about this point to produce a more accurate estimate.

Perfusion

Perfusion can be determined from a first-pass study following a rapid bolus of contrast medium. Details of the derivation of the perfusion algorithm can be found in Chapter 4. The method described by Miles *et al.* [3] uses the simple equation:

$$\text{Perfusion} = \frac{\left[\dfrac{\mathrm{d}c_{\mathrm{t}}}{\mathrm{d}t}\right]_{\max}}{[a(t)]_{\max}}$$

where c_{t} is the tissue enhancement and $a(t)$ is arterial enhancement following administration of the bolus, i.e. perfusion is the ratio of the maximum gradient of the tissue time–density curve and the maximum enhancement of the arterial time–density curve.

The gradient between each pair of scans can be derived using the linear interpolation as follows:

$$\frac{\mathrm{d}c_{\mathrm{t}}}{\mathrm{d}t} = \frac{[c_{\mathrm{t}}]_i - [c_{\mathrm{t}}]_{i-1}}{t_i - t_{i-1}}$$

Cubic interpolation can improve the accuracy of the measurement of the gradient as for the maximum enhancement above.

The maximum arterial enhancement need only be determined once for each sequence of scans. A region of interest should be placed within a suitable vessel and the time–density curve generated used to determine the maximum enhancement. As this value is vital in scaling the perfusion, it is important to avoid any voxels containing a partial volume of tissue as this will reduce the maximum determined.

Permeability and blood volume

Vessel permeability and blood volume can be estimated using measurements taken after the administered contrast has mixed using a model of the transfer of contrast from the intravascular space to the extracellular space. The method was described by Patlak [4] and has been applied to imaging by Ford *et al.* [5] and Bartollini *et al.* [6].

If we assume that the transfer constant from blood to extracellular space is K and that the concentration in the extracellular space is sufficiently low during the procedure that we can ignore the reverse transfer constant, then the tissue concentration c_t is described as a function of K, ϕ_b, the proportion of the voxel or region containing blood, and b the concentration of contrast in the blood.

$$c_t(t) = K\int_0^t b(t)\mathrm{d}t + \phi_b b(t)$$

If we divide through by b then we can derive a graph using

$$\frac{c_t(t)}{b(t)} \text{ and } \frac{\int_0^t b(t)\mathrm{d}t}{b(t)}$$

as y and x respectively.

$$\frac{c_t(t)}{b(t)} = K\frac{\int_0^t b(t)\mathrm{d}t}{b(t)} + \phi_b$$

As described above, the concentrations c_t and b are directly proportional to the enhancement so that

$$\frac{c_t(t)}{b(t)} \text{ and } \frac{\int_0^t b(t)\mathrm{d}t}{b(t)}$$

can be replaced by

$$\frac{E_t(t)}{E_b(t)} \text{ and } \frac{\int_0^t E_b(t)\mathrm{d}t}{E_b(t)}$$

where $E(t)$ is the enhancement, and subscripts t and b refer to tissue and blood, respectively.

This graph should be linear during the period when the assumptions above hold, i.e. from after the contrast has mixed until the concentration in the extracellular space is sufficient for the transfer of contrast back from the extracellular space to the blood to be significant.

Figure 2.12 and Figure 2.13 show time–density curves and a Patlak plot for two regions from a slice though the brain. As can be seen, the Patlak plot is approximately linear for the region between points 2 and 7 and a linear regression can be performed on these points. When generating permeability values for all voxels in an image or for a number of regions, the x-axis values for each point are

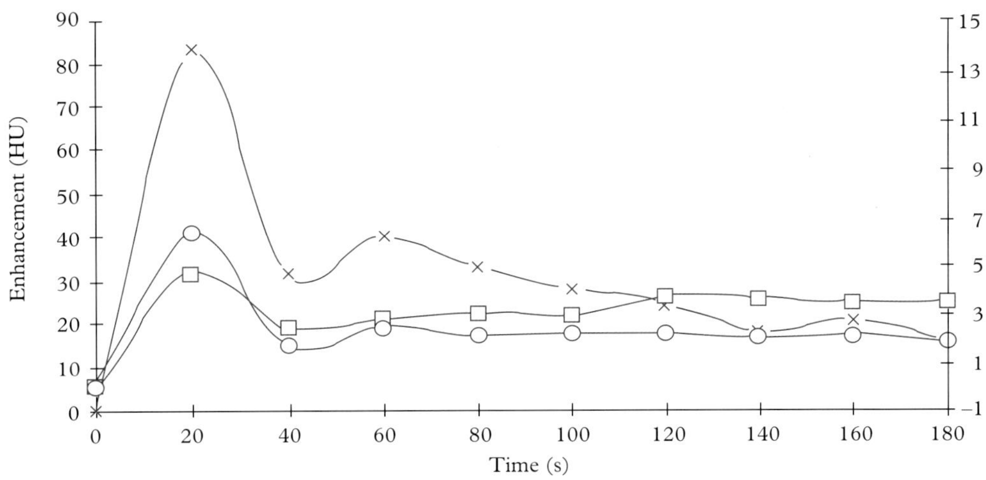

Figure 2.12 Graph showing the time–density curves for a vessel region and two tissue regions in the brain. It is difficult to predict which tissue contains tumour from the time–density curve as shown. × = vessel (left axis); □ = tumour (right axis); ○ = normal (right axis).

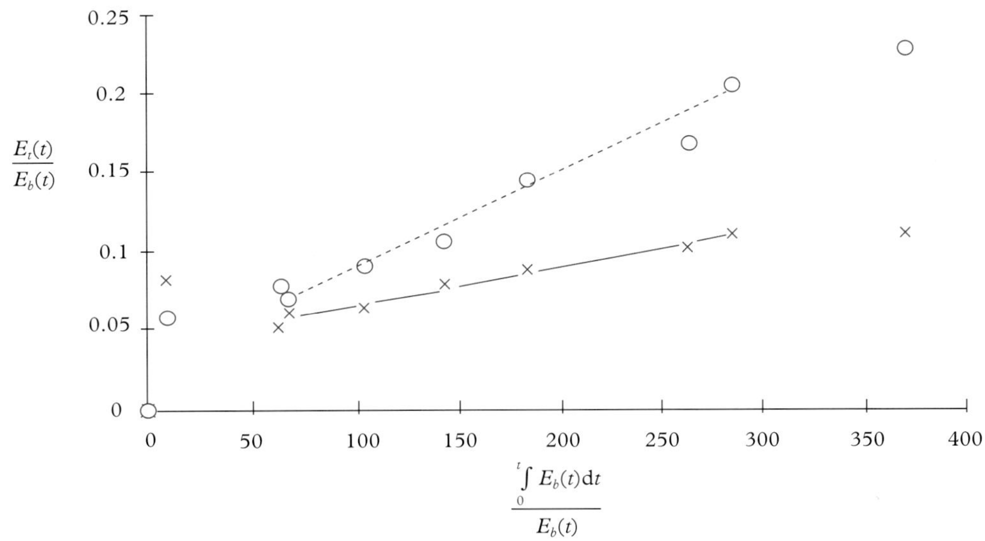

Figure 2.13 Patlak plot from two regions within a brain using the time–density curves in Figure 2.12. The linear fit has been performed for points 2 to 7 (first point is point 0). The blood-volume fraction is derived from the y-intercept of the regression line for each region; the gradient of the line gives the permeability. × = normal; ○ = tumour; ——— = normal; - - - - - - - = tumour.

unchanged throughout the image and this information can be used to optimize the regression calculations.

ESTIMATION OF ERRORS

Effect of noise

The effect of noise on the measurement depends on the analysis algorithm and the interpolation technique. The interpolation techniques used are explained at the end of this chapter (page 25). The presence of noise can produce a systematic bias (i.e. the mean measurement differs from the measurement expected in the absence of noise) and a statistical error in which a variation is seen about the mean measurement.

Except under a few circumstances, there is no simple mathematical relationship between noise amplitude and the errors of measurement. A number of simulations were therefore performed to identify the effect of noise. Time–density curves were taken from a typical patient using a large region of interest (and hence negligible noise) for a number of organs and noise was added using a Gaussian random number generator to simulate noise of a given amplitude. A number of measurements were made for different noise amplitudes and the mean and standard deviation of the values produced were calculated.

In the following examples, 200 simulated measurements were made for each combination of time–density curve, algorithm and noise amplitude unless otherwise stated.

Maximum enhancement

The variation in derivation of maximum enhancement without interpolation was found to be very close to the noise amplitude. This is as would be expected since the maximum in this case depends on only one time–density curve value. If cubic interpolation is used, then the variation in maximum enhancement is reduced — due to averaging over the four points used in the interpolation — until the noise amplitude is sufficient to produce a maximum in a different position which will produce a greater variation. For typical noise levels, the mean value of maximum enhancement varies little. Table 2.1 shows the mean and variation of maximum enhancement values derived from an aortic time–density curve.

Perfusion

Three situations were considered for perfusion measurements: zero perfusion where all measurements in the time–density curve are zero, low perfusion as is found in the liver and high perfusion as found in the cortex of the kidneys. As described above, the perfusion value is the ratio of the maximum gradient for the tissue time–density curve and the maximum enhancement in the arterial time–density curve. As the same value for arterial maximum is used for all calculations on a dataset, this produces a scaling effect on all measurements but does not

	Linear interpolation		Cubic interpolation	
Noise amplitude (standard deviation)	Estimated maximum enhancement (HU)	Error in estimate (standard deviation, HU)	Estimated maximum enhancement (HU)	Error in estimate (standard deviation, HU)
0	227.2	0.00	238.2	0.00
1	227.3	1.06	238.3	0.81
2	227.4	2.17	238.2	1.41
4	227.6	3.78	239.9	5.10

Table 2.1
The variation in estimated maximum enhancement with noise using linear and cubic interpolation; 200 repeats were performed for each noise level

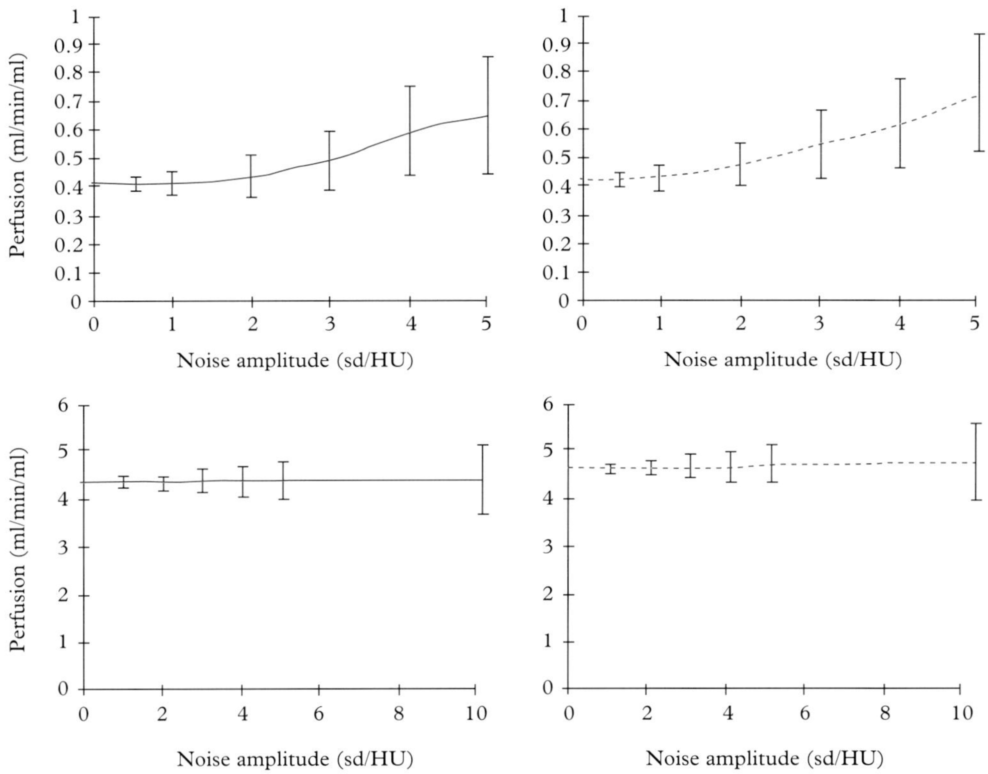

Figure 2.14
Plots of the variation of estimated perfusion as a function of noise amplitude showing mean and standard deviation of the estimated values from 200 iterations. (*Top*) Perfusion estimated from a typical liver time–density curve; linear interpolation on left and cubic interpolation on right. (*Bottom*) Perfusion estimated from the kidney cortex. sd = standard deviation.

affect comparisons within the dataset. Variation within the dataset depends only upon the estimation of the maximum gradient. If linear interpolation is used then the maximum gradient depends on two measurements only. However, if the difference between subsequent values is low compared with the noise, the maximum gradient can be erroneously estimated at the wrong position. The cubic interpolation depends on four measurements and could be expected to be even more sensitive to noise.

As can be seen in Figure 2.14, the mean value of perfusion increases with noise amplitude after a threshold which depends on the amplitude of the true maximum gradient. Figure 2.15 shows the range of values produced from 10 000 estimates using the linear and cubic interpolation on a typical liver time–density curve. For the zero perfusion case, any noise will produce a positive gradient and the perfusion calculated increases linearly with noise amplitude. If noise standard deviation is 2 HU, the apparent perfusion will be 0.18 ± 0.08 ml/min/ml for the linear interpolation and 0.22 ± 0.10 ml/min/ml for the cubic interpolation.

These results have important implications, particularly for the estimation of perfusion in small regions and for voxels. If we assume that typical noise levels for liver measurement give a standard deviation of 4 HU then:

1. Voxels with no perfusion will still give rise to an average perfusion of 0.36 ml/min/ml or 0.44 ml/min/ml depending on interpolation — this is comparable with the expected perfusion value.

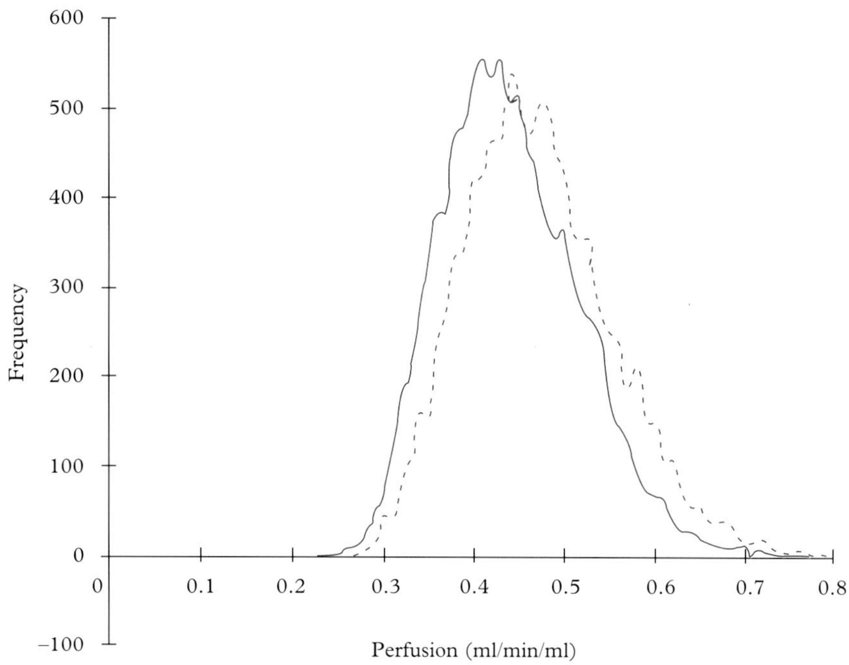

Figure 2.15
Histograms showing the range of perfusion values derived for a noise standard deviation of 2 HU from a typical liver time–density curve.
——— = Linear interpolation;
- - - - - - - = cubic interpolation.

2. The estimated perfusion in liver voxels will be raised approximately 40% above the true value.
3. The error in measurement of perfusion in the liver voxels will be approximately 25% (standard deviation).

If we use smoothing of degree one then the noise standard deviation is reduced by a factor of two and the equivalent figures are:

1. Voxels with no perfusion will still give rise to an average perfusion of 0.18 ml/min/ml or 0.22 ml/min/ml. This is the equivalent of a low perfusion region within the liver.
2. The estimated perfusion in liver voxels will be not be significantly increased above their true value.
3. The error in measurement of perfusion in the liver voxels will be approximately 10% (standard deviation).

Use of a ROI would be expected to reduce the noise standard deviation by the square root of the number of pixels and hence should reduce the errors above to insignificant proportions for a reasonable-sized region.

Permeability and red-cell volume

As the permeability measurement depends on a linear fit to a number of given points, the effect of noise is particularly difficult to estimate. Figure 2.16 shows

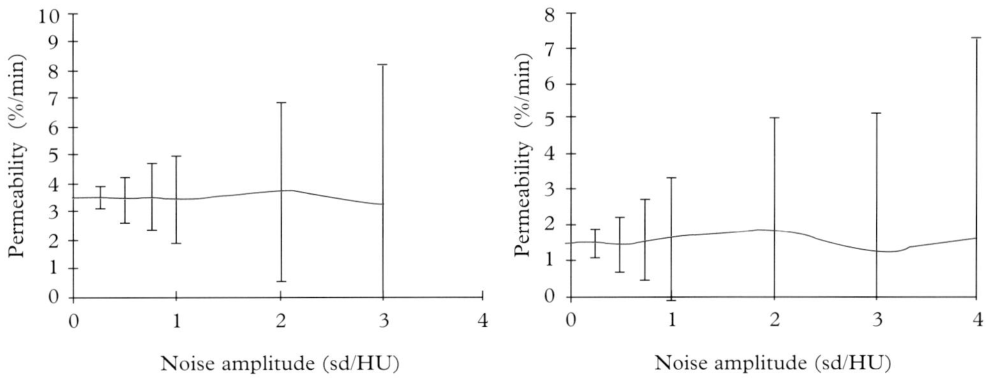

Figure 2.16
Plots of the variation of estimated permeability as a function of noise amplitude showing mean and standard deviation (sd) of the estimated values from 200 iterations. The left shows the estimated errors for a brain tumour time–density curve, the right shows a normal brain time–density curve (see Figure 2.13).

the variation of estimated permeability with noise for two typical time–density curves. From this graph it is apparent that the Patlak technique amplifies noise within the time–density curve and a great deal of smoothing is required to produce images of acceptable quality. There is, however, less variation in the mean estimated value than in the case of perfusion. For quantitation purposes, it is recommended that ROIs be used.

PRESENTATION OF DATA

It is very important when displaying the results of functional imaging to make clear the conditions under which the calculations were performed. In particular, any threshold filters and any smoothing applied should be quoted. For regions of interest, an indication of the number of voxels included can indicate the statistical significance of the measurements.

The production of images from processing of time–density curves for each voxel can be a very useful means of presentation of the results. Our preference has been to use a false colour scale as opposed to a grey scale to indicate the value in each voxel for quantitative parameters. This allows easy identification of regions of similar perfusion as the eye can match colours more easily than matching grey levels but can lead to the creation of apparent contours at the borders between colours, and caution must be applied to be consistent in the windowing used when comparing images.

As demonstrated above, functional parameters derived from single voxels may have a significant error attached to them and more importantly, may give a greater value than would a larger region of interest with reduced noise. For this reason, it is very important that quantitation of regions is performed by generating a time–density curve from the raw data using the region as a boundary and then performing the calculation on this time–density curve. Averaging the result from a number of individual time–density curves for each voxel can lead to a significant bias in the results.

SUMMARY

In summary, the following steps are required for the production of functional images from CT data:

1. Generation of a single-location dynamic sequence of slices. Most CT systems will allow this with a fixed time delay; some allow the interscan delay to be varied throughout the acquisition.
2. Transfer to a workstation for processing. Very few, if any, CT systems have any ability to produce functional images beyond the simple maximum enhancement and time to maximum images so the images must be transferred to an alternative workstation. Means for this transfer vary for different machines although DICOM 3.0 now defines a standard to which all manufacturers should now comply.
3. Access to the images from a functional imaging program. This can be the most difficult step as it depends on the data format of the images and the design of the workstation and will require a high level of technical support.
4. A means for processing the images using the algorithms described here. This must be coded using a fast, compiled language and there are few tools available which perform the manipulations required. If it is possible to transfer the images to a nuclear medicine or positron emission tomography (PET) workstation, then it is likely some or all of the required tools will be available.

Consideration must be given to the following:

1. Some of the algorithms described are sensitive to noise variations in the time–density curves produced — steps should be taken to keep noise below levels at which a bias will be introduced to the measurements.
2. In general, parameters derived from a single voxel will not produce accurate quantitation — although suitable for the production of images, quantitation should be derived from time–density curves generated from a larger ROI.
3. Care must be taken not to include vessels, bone or air within the ROI for a tissue as this will bias the measurement of certain parameters. A threshold filter can be used to eliminate these voxels.

A computer program running under Microsoft Windows™ has been produced by the author for the University of Cambridge Department of Radiology which implements all of the above algorithms. It will accept input in a DICOM or ACR/NEMA format and has a general purpose algorithm for the input of any, uncompressed data format. It can be obtained from the author via e-mail (*mike@radiol.cam.ac.uk*) and will be on display at the University of Cambridge Department of Radiology WWW site (*http://www.his.path.cam.ac.uk/rad/radiol.html*).

APPENDIX

Interpolation of time–density curve data

The time–density curve created from a dynamic series contains a number of discrete measurements. From this time–density curve, four parameters are required for perfusion measurements: the maximum enhancement, the time of maximum enhancement, the maximum gradient and the time of maximum gradient. It is assumed that noise is negligible and hence the interpolated curve should pass through all points.

Figure 2.10 compares two interpolation techniques. The simplest method of interpolation is linear interpolation. The function is considered to continue in a straight line between points. This obviously can underestimate the maximum enhancement if the maximum occurs between two measurements and will lead to a limited range of time values. An interpolation technique commonly used in dynamic CT is to apply the cubic spline. This is based on a draughtsman's tool but essentially involves the fitting of a cubic equation to each series of four points such that the slope and curvature of two joining cubics are matched. This technique requires a great deal of calculation and hence a simplified algorithm has been developed.

An initial analysis is made of the curve using linear interpolation and the position of the maximum or maximum gradient is determined. If the point is at one of the two ends (this rarely occurs in practice) then the linear interpolated value is returned, otherwise a cubic is fitted to pass through the four points surrounding the position of the maximum or maximum gradient. This is equivalent to using the cubic spline but requires less calculation. Once the cubic has been derived, the required analysis parameters can be derived directly from the cubic equation.

The cubic will be of the form:

$$y = a_0 + a_1 t + a_2 t^2 + a_3 t^3 = p(t) \tag{1}$$

and from four points, four simultaneous equations can be derived and hence the four unknowns a_0, a_1, a_2 and a_3 can be derived:

$$a_0 = -\sum_i \left(\frac{y_i \prod_{i \neq j} t_j}{m_i} \right) \tag{2}$$

$$a_1 = \sum_i \left(\frac{y_i \sum_{i \neq j} \sum_{i \neq k} t_j t_k}{m_i} \right) \tag{3}$$

$$a_2 = -\sum_i \left(\frac{y_i \sum_{i \neq j} t_j}{m_i} \right) \tag{4}$$

$$a_3 = -\sum_i \frac{y_i}{m_i} \tag{5}$$

where

$$m_i = \prod_{i \neq j} (t_i - t_j) \tag{6}$$

The maximum, $y_{\max}$ occurs at $t_{y\ \max}$ when $\frac{\mathrm{d}}{\mathrm{d}t} p(t) = 0$ and $\frac{\mathrm{d}^2}{\mathrm{d}t^2} p(t) < 0$:

$$t_{y\ \max} = \frac{-2a_2 \pm \sqrt{4a_2^2 - 12a_1a_3}}{2a_1} \tag{7}$$

$$y_{\max} = p(t_{y\ \max}) \text{ if } a_2 + 6a_3 < 0. \tag{8}$$

The maximum gradient $g_{\max}$ occurs at $t_{g\ \max}$:

$$t_{g\ \max} = -\frac{a_2}{3a_3} \text{ if } a_3 < 0 \tag{9}$$

$$g_{\max} = \frac{\mathrm{d}^2}{\mathrm{d}t^2} p(t_{g\ \max}) \tag{10}$$

The gamma-variate function

The gamma-variate function is often used to describe the shape of the bolus as it appears in the time–density curve. The form is as follows:

$$c(t) = k(t - t_\mathrm{a})^\alpha \mathrm{e}^{\frac{-(t - t_\alpha)}{\beta}} \tag{11}$$

k defines the magnitude of the curve; α and β define the shape. Note the function is undefined for values of t below t_a, the time of arrival of the bolus. The shape is the same as that for the gamma-distribution function used in statistics.

Figure 2.11 shows a selection of gamma-variate curves. Non-iterative determination of the best-fit gamma variate for a given time–density curve is not simple. The following shows one method for the determination of k, α and β, assuming t_a is known. First, logarithms are taken of both sides of the equations

$$\ln(c(t)) = \ln(k) + \alpha \ln(t - t_\mathrm{a}) - \frac{(t - t_\mathrm{a})}{\beta} \tag{12}$$

this can be rewritten thus:

$$y_i = \mu + a_1x_{1i} + a_2x_{2i} \tag{13}$$

where

$$y_i = \ln(c(t)),\quad a_1 = \alpha,\quad a_2 = -\frac{1}{\beta},\quad \mu = \ln(k),\quad x_{1i} = \ln(t_i - t_\mathrm{a}) \text{ and } x_{2i} = (t_i - t_\mathrm{a})$$

For a least-squares fit of a gamma variate to a given time–density curve, we must minimize the equation:

$$\sum_i w_i(y_i - \mu - a_1x_{1i} - a_2x_{2i})^2 \tag{14}$$

w_i is a weighting function for each point in the time–density curve and y_i x_{1i} and x_{2i} are derived from the time–density curve data points. If we partially differentiate Equation (14) with respect to μ, a_1 a_2 we produce the following equations:

$$\frac{\partial c}{\partial \mu} = \sum_i w_i \left(y_i - \mu - a_1 x_{1i} - a_2 x_{2i} \right) = 0 \tag{15}$$

$$\frac{\partial c}{\partial a_1} = \sum_i w_i \left(x_{1i} y_i - \mu x_{1i} - a_1 x_{1i}^2 - a_2 x_{2i} x_{1i} \right) = 0 \tag{16}$$

$$\frac{\partial c}{\partial a_2} = \sum_i w_i \left(x_{2i} y_i - \mu x_{2i} - a_1 x_{1i} x_{2i} - a_2 x_{2i}^2 \right) = 0 \tag{17}$$

These can be rearranged to:

$$\mu \sum w_i + a_1 \sum w_i x_{1i} + a_2 \sum w_i x_{2i} = \sum y_i w_i \tag{18}$$

$$\mu \sum w_i x_{1i} + a_1 \sum w_i x_{1i}^2 + a_2 \sum w_i x_{1i} x_{2i} = \sum y_i w_i x_{1i} \tag{19}$$

$$\mu \sum w_i x_{2i} + a_1 \sum w_i x_{1i} x_{2i} + a_2 \sum w_i x_{2i}^2 = \sum y_i w_i x_{2i} \tag{20}$$

It can be seen that these equations can be expressed in the form:

$$\begin{pmatrix} A_{11}\mu & A_{12}a_1 & A_{13}a_2 \\ A_{21}\mu & A_{22}a_1 & A_{23}a_2 \\ A_{31}\mu & A_{32}a_1 & A_{33}a_2 \end{pmatrix} = \begin{pmatrix} B_1 \\ B_2 \\ B_3 \end{pmatrix}, \begin{matrix} A_{12} = A_{21} \\ A_{23} = A_{32} \\ A_{13} = A_{31} \end{matrix} \tag{21}$$

which can be solved using matrix algebra using:

$$\begin{pmatrix} \mu \\ a_1 \\ a_2 \end{pmatrix} = A^{-1}B \tag{22}$$

This form of the solution is suitable for use in a computer algorithm. Since the matrix A does not depend on the enhancement values, it can be calculated in advance for image processing.

In most cases, the value t_a, the bolus arrival time, is not known. If the noise is sufficiently low, then the time at which the time–density curve rises above zero is a reasonable estimate of the arrival time. Where the arrival time cannot be estimated, an iterative process can be used to determine the best-fit value of t_a but this is processor intensive.

Some features of the gamma variate

The differential with respect to time is as follows:

$$\frac{\mathrm{d}c(t)}{\mathrm{d}t} = -\frac{k}{\beta}(t - t_a)^{\alpha} e^{-\frac{(t-t_a)}{\beta}} + \alpha k (t - t_a)^{(\alpha - 1)} e^{-\frac{(t-t_a)}{\beta}} = \left(\frac{\alpha}{(t - t_a)} - \frac{1}{\beta} \right) c(t) \tag{23}$$

and hence the maximum occurs when $\mathrm{d}c(t)/\mathrm{d}t = 0$ when $\alpha\beta = t - t_a$.

Thus:

$$t_{\text{peak}} = t_a + \alpha\beta \tag{24}$$

$$c_{\text{peak}} = k(\alpha\beta)^{\alpha}e^{-\alpha} \tag{25}$$

The area under the curve can be derived by rearranging the integral. Substitute $\tau = t - t_a, \alpha = n - 1, \tau = \beta x$.

$$c(t) = k\tau^{\alpha}e^{\frac{-\tau}{\beta}} \tag{26}$$

Thus:

$$k\int_0^{\infty}\tau^{\alpha}e^{\frac{-\tau}{\beta}}\,d\tau = k\int_0^{\infty}(\beta x)^{n-1}e^{-x}\beta dx = k\beta^n\int_0^{\infty}x^{n-1}e^{-x}dx = k\beta^n\Gamma(n) \tag{27}$$

Summarizing:

$$\int_{t_a}^{\infty}c(t)dt = k\beta^{\alpha+1}\Gamma(\alpha+1) \tag{28}$$

where $\Gamma(n)$ is the gamma function which reduces to the factorial for integral values of α. Tables and subroutines for the derivation of the gamma function are commonly available.

REFERENCES

1. Blomley, M.J., Coulden, R., Bufkin, C., Lipton, M.J. and Dawson, P. (1993) Contrast bolus dynamic computed tomography for the measurement of solid organ perfusion. *Investigative Radiology*, **28**(Suppl 5), S72–7; discussion S78.
2. Miyakawa, E. (1993) The assessment of tumor blood flow factors using dynamic CT — a comparison with positron emission tomography (in Japanese). *Nippon Igaku Hoshasen Gakkai Zasshi (Nippon Acta Radiologica)*, **53**(3), 297–307.
3. Miles, K.A., Hayball, M. and Dixon, A.K. (1991) Colour perfusion imaging: a new application of computed tomography. *Lancet*, **337**(8742), 643–645.
4. Patlak, C.S., Blasberg, R.G. and Fensternmacher, J.D. (1983) Graphical evolution of blood to brain transfer constants from multijob time uptake data. *Journal of Cerebral Blood Flow and Metabolism*, **3**, 1–7.
5. Ford, J.M., Miles, K.A., Hayball, M.P., Bearcroft, P.W., Blechen, N.M. and Osborn, C.S. (1996) A simplified technique for measurement of blood–brain barrier permeability using CT: preliminary results of the effect of RMP-7. Quantitative Imaging Oncology, Proceedings of 19th LH Gray Conference *British Journal of Radiology*, p. 1–5.
6. Bartolini, A., Gasparetto, B., Furlan, M., Primavera, A., Amore, R., Sullo, L. and Trivelli, G. (1994) Functional circulation and blood–brain permeability images by angio CT in the assessment of cerebral ischemia. *Computerized Medical Imaging & Graphics*, **18**(3), 151–161.

Chapter 3

CONTRAST AGENTS AS TRACERS

P. Dawson

Medical imaging has made enormous advances since its origins with the discovery of X-rays by Röntgen in 1895. In addition to the inevitable increase in sophistication of the basic X-ray tubes, power supplies and film–screen combinations, the advent of small computers has given us computed tomography (CT). Further, the latter part of the first century of medical imaging has been marked by the introduction of powerful non-X-ray imaging technologies, ultrasound (US) and magnetic resonance imaging (MRI). At this, the beginning of its second century, medical imaging is poised on the brink of a digital revolution with all that this implies for radiation dosimetry, X-ray image acquisition, storage, retrieval, transmission and manipulation of data. Computer power has restored the third dimension to the once strictly two-dimensional X-ray imaging. One facet of the digital revolution, underemphasized perhaps because not widely appreciated, is that the acquisition of data in digital form holds the potential for quantitative measurements. Combined with the fact that the modern technologies are capable of fast repetition of images/datasets, this opens up the possibility of quantitative measurement of parameters of physiological significance; that is to say functional/ physiological imaging becomes possible.

The history of radiology has been the history of constant improvements in the quality of anatomical demonstration in medical images for diagnostic purposes and the radiologist, as discussed in Chapter 1, has traditionally been interested in anatomy rather than function. A shift to physiological imaging represents a significant role extension.

The very earliest development in the efforts to improve X-ray anatomical images came within one month of Röntgen's discovery when two groups, one in Vienna [1] and one in Sheffield, England [2], realized the need for, and developed primitive versions of, intravascular contrast enhancing agents (Figure 3.1). A significant part of the subsequent history of radiology has been that of the improvement of the efficacy and safety of such agents [3].

All imaging modalities, including US and MRI, benefit from use of their own specific agents but we are concerned here with the X-ray contrast-enhancing agents. These are iodine-containing organic compound solutions which modify contrast simply by increasing X-ray absorption differentially in one tissue as compared with another or in abnormal tissues as compared with normal. It

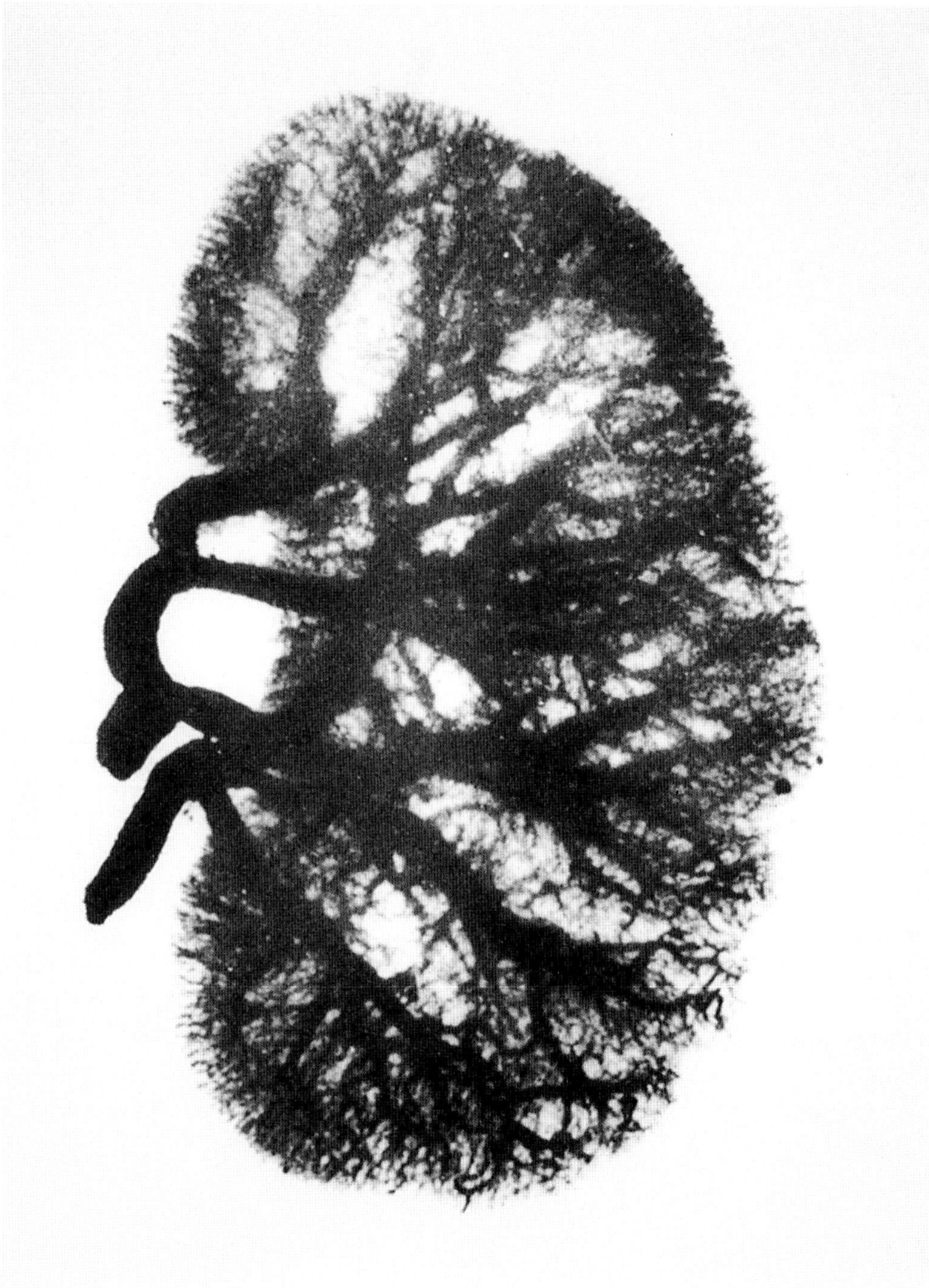

Figure 3.1
Perhaps the very earliest contrast enhanced study on a cadaver kidney (January 1896) [2].

requires little imagination to see, in principle, how digital data from a series of, say, CT images acquired following a bolus injection of such a contrast-enhancing agent might be exploited to derive useful physiological information. In short, contrast agents may be used not simply for their usual design purpose but as 'tracers' in bolus tracking experiments. As will be discussed, CT is a particularly useful technology with which to exploit these ideas because of the special linear characteristics of the CT N°.

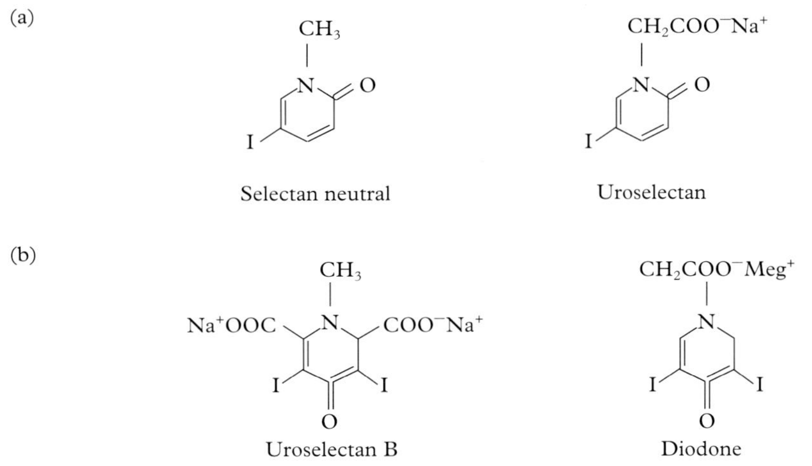

Figure 3.2
The (a) mono- and (b) diodinated pyridone compounds used until the early 1950s.

X-RAY CONTRAST-ENHANCING AGENTS

While a variety of heavy elements, such as gadolinium [4], might be used as X-ray contrast agents, the element exploited in all commercial products is iodine. The first clinically effective agents, dating from the late 1920s were iodinated pyridones (Figure 3.2) [3,5]. From the 1950s, the benzene ring replaced the pyridine ring in the first major improvement in both efficacy and tolerance (Figure 3.3) [3,5]. From the 1980s, radiologists have had at their disposal a group of highly effective, very well tolerated and markedly safer 'low osmolality' non-ionic agents [6,7] with considerable advantages over their predecessors (Figure 3.4). The very latest development, the non-ionic dimers, iotrolan and iodixanol [8,9] (Figure 3.5), probably represent the end of the development road for this kind of agent in that the osmolality is even further reduced from a level of about threefold the plasma osmolality in the non-ionic monomers to that of plasma, while the intrinsic chemotoxicity remains as low as in the non-ionic

Figure 3.3
The iodinated benzoic acid derivatives (ionic agents) introduced in the 1950s.

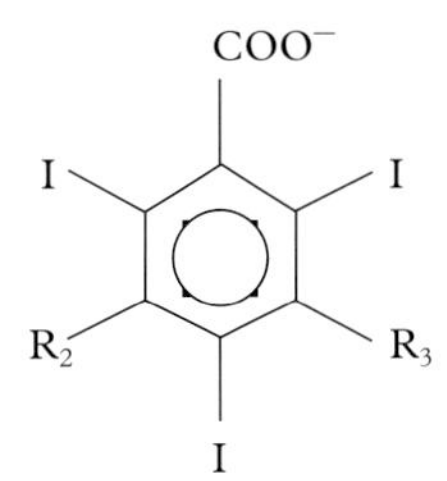

R_2	R_3	Proper name	Commercial name
H	$NHCOCH_3$	Acetrizoate	Urokon, Diaginol
CH_3CONH	$NHCOCH_3$	Diatrizoate	Urografin, Hypaque
CH_3CONH	$CONHCH_3$	Iothalamate	Conray
CH_3CONH	$NCOCH_3$ (N–CH_3)	Metrizoate	Isopaque, Triosil

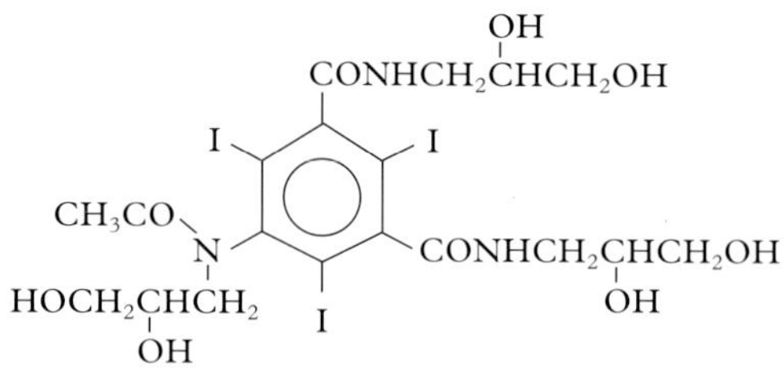

Figure 3.4
A typical non-ionic monomeric agent. Although termed 'low osmolality', such agents are still some threefold plasma osmolality at their higher concentrations.

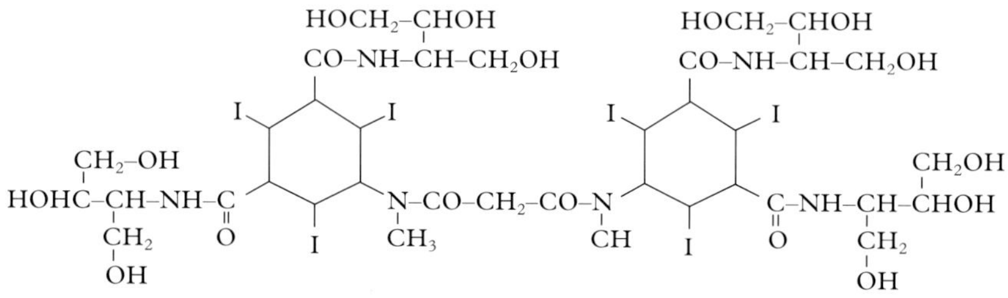

Figure 3.5
The non-ionic dimer, iotrolan. This, and its counterpart, iodixanol, are iso-osmolar with plasma in all formulations while retaining the characteristic low chemotoxicity of the non-ionic monomers.

monomers [8,9]. Osmolalities are shown in Figure 3.6. As will be discussed below in more detail, it is important that any tracer substance used to measure a physiological index should not significantly alter that index. High tolerance, in every sense, is therefore the *sine qua non* in this application.

PHARMACOLOGY AND PHARMACOKINETICS

Pharmacology

These agents have no pharmacology in the conventional sense. They are stable and inert, undergoing no breakdown or metabolism, and being excreted unchanged by passive glomerular filtration without any significant active tubular secretion or reabsorption. They do, however, to a varying degree, exert a number of effects on biochemistry and physiology which are mediated principally by a combination of hyperosmolality and chemotoxicity [3,10–17], though incipients in some formulations may also have their own effects. The so-called 'low osmolality' non-ionic monomeric agents are still some threefold plasma osmolality at concentrations typically used clinically [3] and so, in higher doses, still exert significant osmolality-related effects such as smooth muscle relaxation [3,18], fluid shifts [15], vasopressin release [16,17], red-cell rigidification [13], basophil histamine release [11] and cardiac failure [19].

The non-ionic dimers are iso-osmolar with plasma and exert no such osmolality-related effects. However, all X-ray contrast agents have an intrinsic toxicity, a 'chemotoxicity', which is a function of chemical structure and is mediated by non-specific hydrophobic and (in ionic agents) Coulomb interactions with structural and functional proteins [14,20]. This is a phenomenon seen only because of the, by any standards, high doses of these materials used clinically.

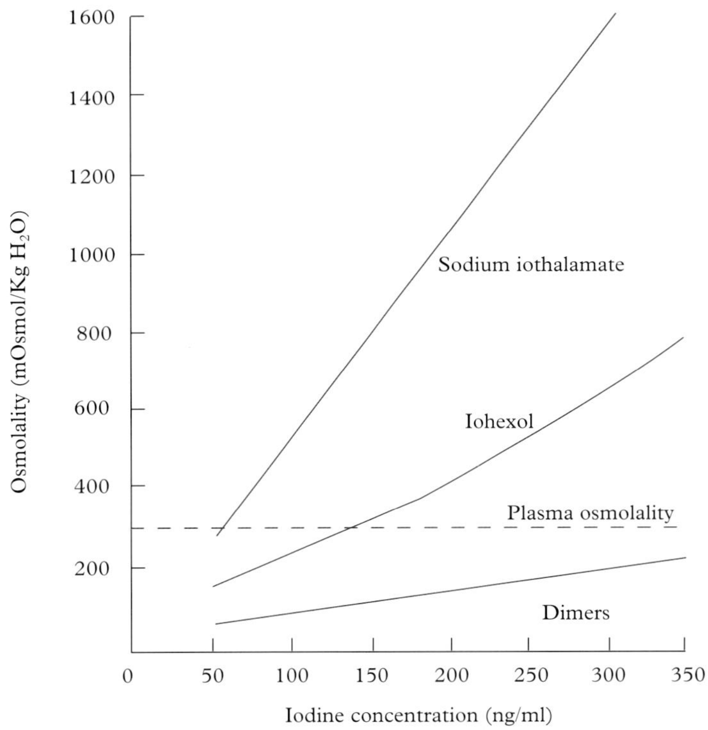

Figure 3.6
The osmolalities of different contrast-agent types, ionic monomeric, non-ionic monomeric and the dimers as a function of iodine concentration. In commercial formulations the dimers are adjusted to iso-osmolality with plasma by addition of electrolytes.

The non-ionic agents, monomeric and dimeric, are electrically neutral and therefore exert no Coulomb effects and are highly hydrophilic, the hydrophobic benzene–iodine core of the molecules being (variably) effectively shielded by hydrophilic substituents [14,20].

The non-ionic monomers and dimers combine low osmolality with low chemotoxicity to yield much diminished effects on all physiological and biochemical parameters and, consequently, better all-round tolerance [8,9,14]. Some specific effects of contrast agents, particularly their use in functional imaging, will be discussed later.

Pharmacokinetics

The pharmacokinetics of these small molecules are relatively simple. They may be described by a two-compartment model (Figure 3.7), plasma and extracellular extravascular (interstitial) spaces representing the two compartments [21–24]. They do not to any significant extent enter the intracellular space.

On injection, mixing in the plasma and leak across blood-vessel walls into the interstitium rapidly occurs. Passive filtration also begins immediately at first-pass. In the simplified pharmacokinetic model it is assumed that complete and uniform mixing in the plasma occurs before, at arbitrary time $t = 0$, transfer to the interstitium and renal filtration occur. In this case we may write,

$$p(t) = Ae^{-\lambda_1 t} + Be^{-\lambda_2 t} \tag{1}$$

$$C_{\text{is}}(t) = C(e^{-\lambda_2 t} - e^{-\lambda_1 t}) \tag{2}$$

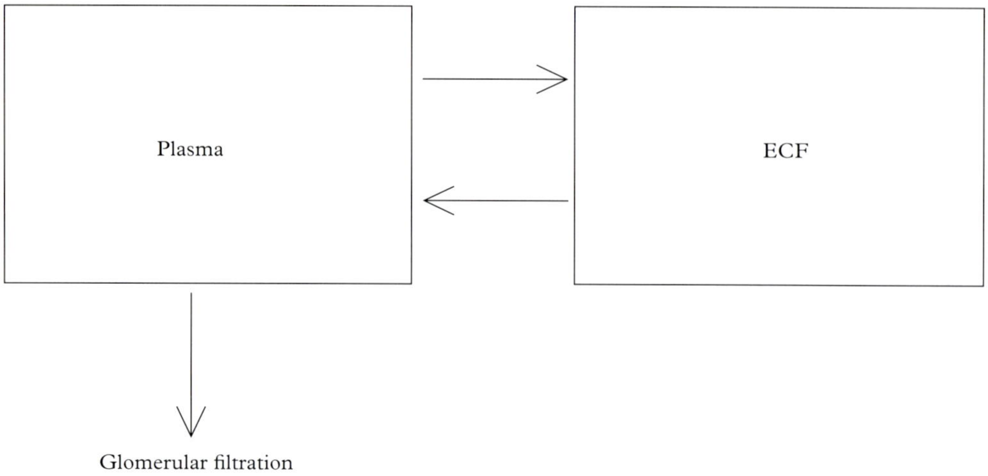

Figure 3.7
The two-compartment pharmacokinetic model. The compartments are plasma and interstitium (ECF).

where $p(t)$ is the plasma concentration and $C_{is}(t)$ the interstitium concentration. A, B, C are constants, where $A + B$ is the total dose given/plasma volume. $\lambda_1 >> \lambda_2$, so the second term comes to dominate later.

If a substantial load of such an agent is considered to raise the plasma osmolality it is quite easy to build into these equations a new rate constant describing the osmotically-driven fluid shifts from interstitium to plasma and from circulating cells to plasma.

Since $\lambda_1 >> \lambda_2$, at later times,

$$p(t) \sim Be^{-\lambda t} \tag{3}$$

So

$$\ell n p(t) \sim -\lambda_2 t + \ell n B \tag{4}$$

A semi-log plot of $\ell n p(t)$ versus t will at later times yield a straight line of gradient $-\lambda_2$ and intercept on the ordinate $\ell n B$ (Figure 3.8).

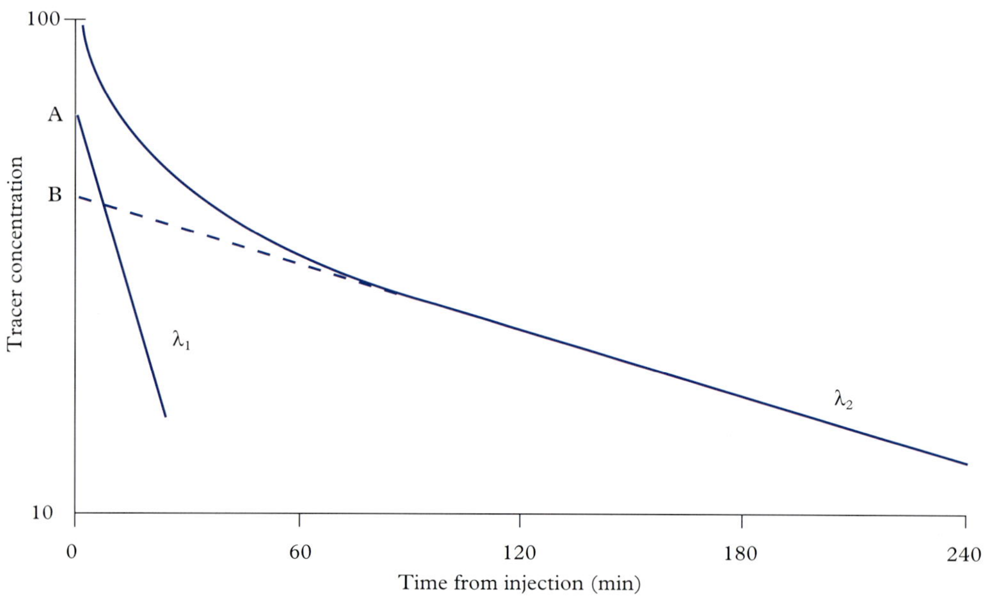

Figure 3.8
A semi-log plot of plasma concentration against time. The later part of the curve is approximately linear.

Dawson and Blomley [21] have shown that in an n-compartment model, $\lambda_n =$ GFR/V_β when V_β is the value of $V_\beta(t)$ at late times (GFR = glomerular filtration rate). $V_\beta(t)$ is the ratio of total amount of tracer in the body and plasma concentration. For a pure extracellular fluid (ECF) agent, $V_\beta \approx V_{\text{ECF}}$. In the more sophisticated model, a semi-log plot as described will still tend to a straight line with slope $-\lambda_n$.

Dawson and Blomley have further shown that the central volume theorem may be adapted to describe the transit of contrast agent through the body [21]. The central volume is taken to be ECF volume and 'flow' is taken to be GFR. This leads to an interpretation of λ_2 as GFR/ECF. This is a most fundamental measure of GFR since one of the central roles of this aspect of renal function is the modulation of ECF volume. Values of $p(t)$ may be obtained by taking blood samples and, after spinning down and separating the samples, using X-ray fluorescence analysis to measure plasma iodine (or gadolinium) concentrations. Dedicated and easy-to-use equipment is available for this task and the technique represents a viable approach to the measurement of renal function incidental to any examination involving contrast administration. Alternatively, it may be performed by the injection of only 25 ml or so of a safe non-ionic agent specifically for the purpose.

Unfortunately, this classical, simplified analysis ignores the brief but crucial period following contrast agent bolus injection which is so important in modern fast imaging whether anatomical or, as discussed below, physiological imaging is the aim. The difficulty lies in mathematically modelling the process of mixing in the plasma, contrast leak into the interstitium and osmotically driven fluid shifts in, say, the first minute after bolus injection. All these events occur simultaneously. The difficulties are clearly reflected in the dearth in the literature of good early pharmacokinetic data for contrast agents, a problem which has been discussed in some detail elsewhere by Blomley and Dawson [25].

These difficulties notwithstanding, it is possible to obtain a great deal of physiological information from rapid sequence image datasets taken during this early phase and this theme forms the basis of this book.

MODE OF ACTION OF X-RAY CONTRAST AGENTS AND ROLE AS TRACERS

The mechanism of action of X-ray contrast media is very simple; the iodine absorbs X-rays and increases the X-ray absorption coefficient in any region of interest containing contrast molecules, whether these are intravascular or extravascular. In CT, the absorption coefficient in any region of interest (ROI), from whole organ down to pixel level, is expressed as a CT N°.

$$\text{CT N}^\circ = K\frac{\mu_\text{p} - \mu_\text{w}}{\mu_\text{w}}$$

where μ_p is the mean absorption coefficient of the pixel, μ_w that of water and where K is a scaling factor usually chosen to be 1000.

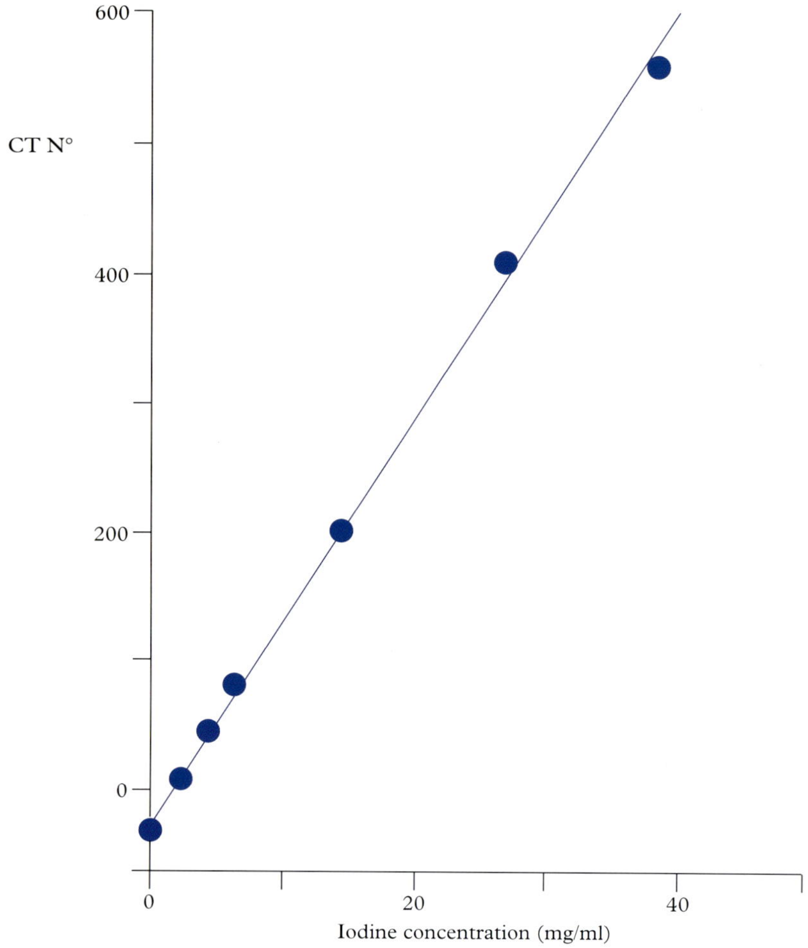

Figure 3.9
CT N° versus iodine-concentration. Data obtained from measurements on a Siemens Somaton Plus. Constant of proportionality is ~ 25 HU per mg/ml iodine.

The beauty of the CT N° is that, if beam hardening and partial volume effects are minimized, it varies linearly with iodine/contrast concentration (Figure 3.9). That is to say, if the precontrast background CT N° in a ROI is subtracted from any postcontrast CT N°, the result is dependably proportional to the iodine concentration in that ROI.

An accurate calibration may easily be made for any individual scanner at a given kVp, but the constant of proportionality is close to 25 HU per mg/ml iodine.

A series of CT datasets following a bolus injection of a contrast agent allows a background-subtracted CT N° versus time curve to be generated for a whole organ or ROI down to pixel level. Such curves are shown in Figures 3.10 to 3.13 for liver, spleen, kidney and aorta.

It is clear that a wealth of, information, usually neglected, is hidden in such curves. The first part of the curves, up to a time less than the minimum transit time through the ROI, contains information on blood flow or, to be more precise, perfusion, in that ROI, since it is blood which carries the tracer into the tissues.

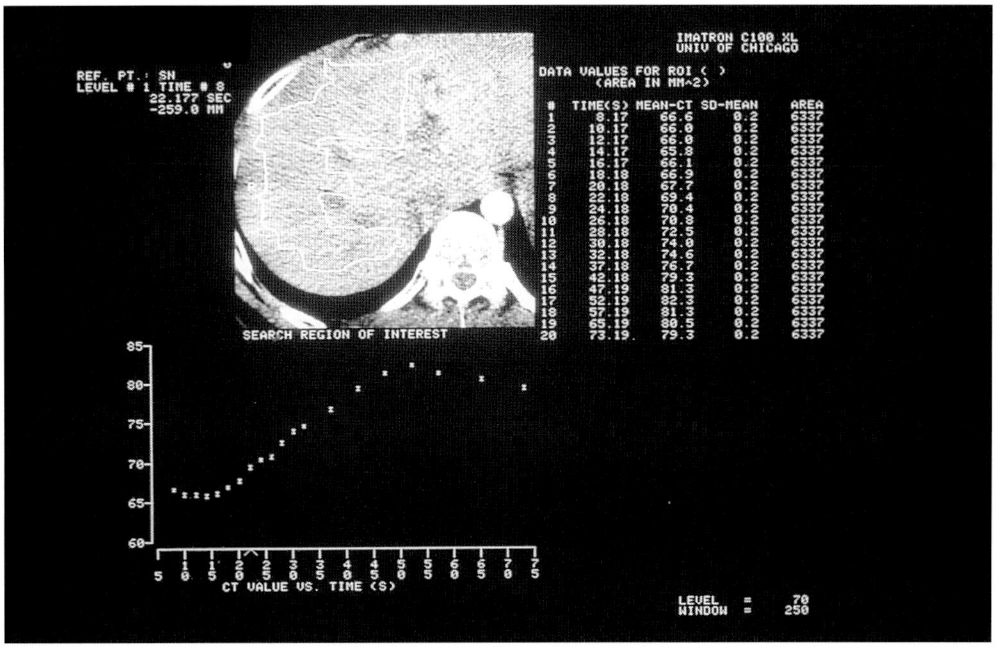

Figure 3.10
Typical liver CT N°–time curve.

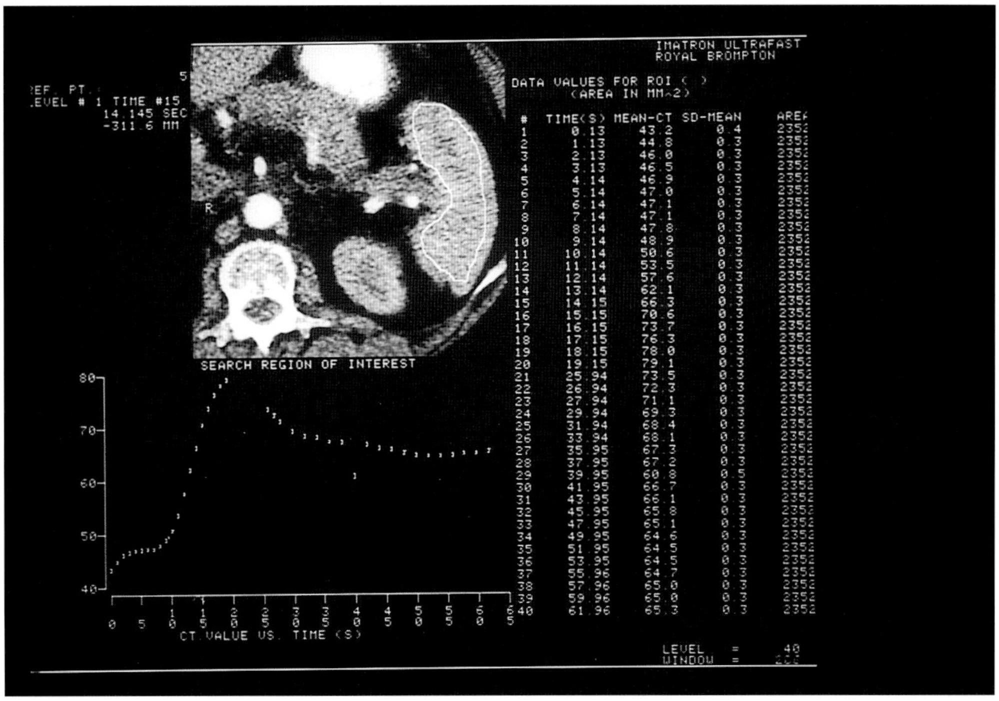

Figure 3.11
Typical splenic CT N°–time curve.

Up to the minimum transit time, the organ is an accumulator or integrator (Figure 3.14). A number of mathematical approaches have been developed to allow calculation of perfusion values from such curves and these are discussed in Chapter 4.

Further, as will be understood from the discussion of pharmacokinetics, these curves also contain hidden information on compartmentalization. The CT N° in

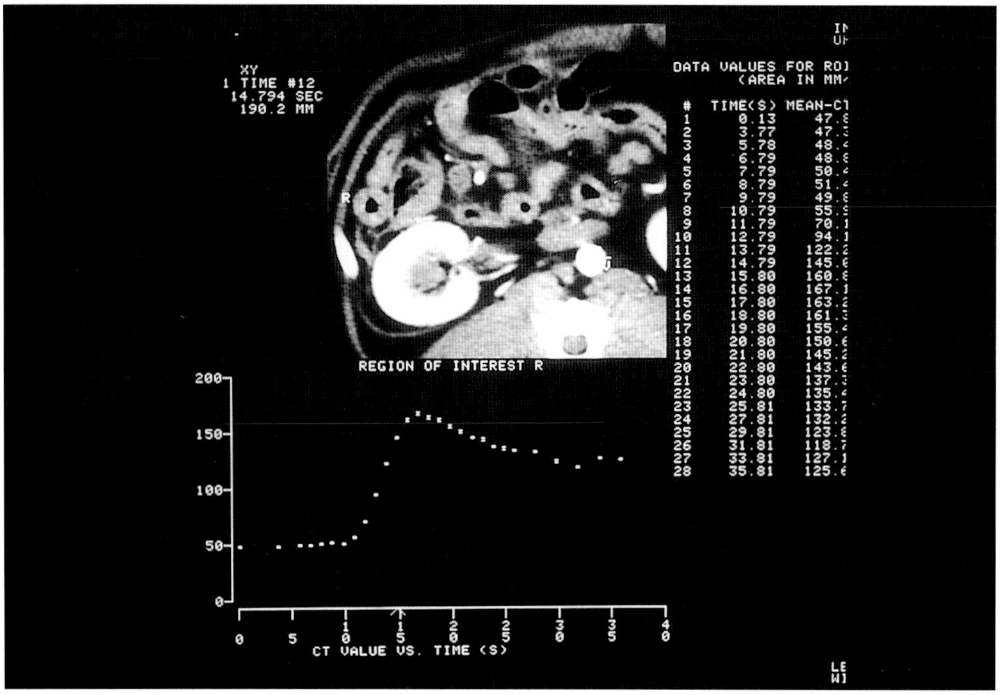

Figure 3.12
Typical renal CT N°–time curve.

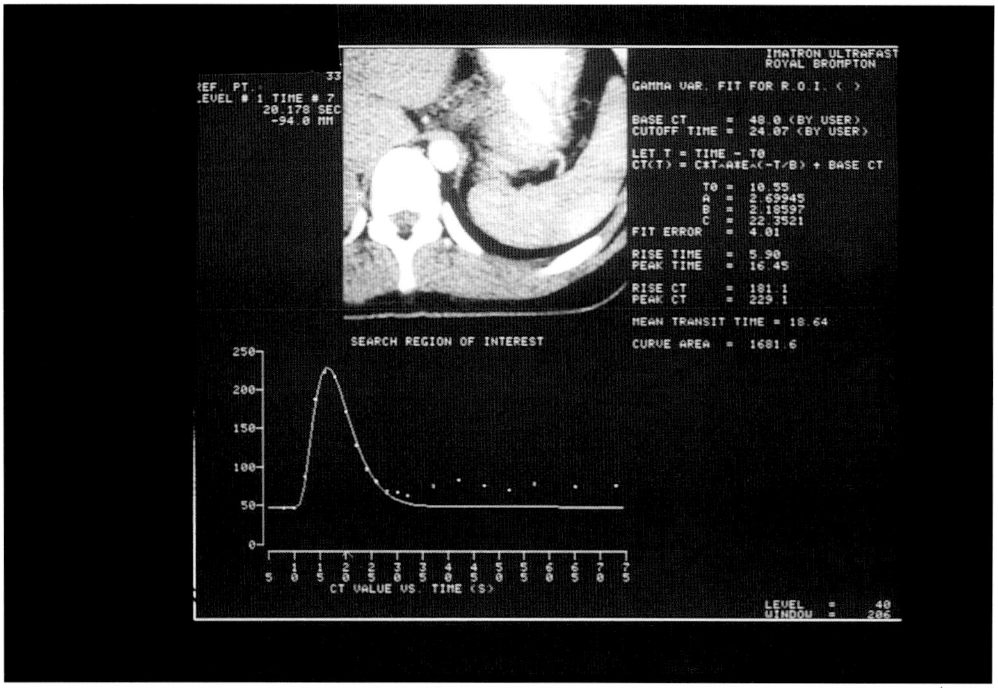

Figure 3.13
Typical aortic CT N°–time curve.

a ROI is the aggregate result of the effects of contrast agent in blood and in interstitium (Figure 3.15). This may be expressed mathematically as follows:

$$c(t) = \phi_{is} C_{is}(t) + \phi_b b(t) \quad (5)$$

where ϕ_b and ϕ_{is} are the proportions of the ROI occupied by blood and interstitium (Figure 3.15)

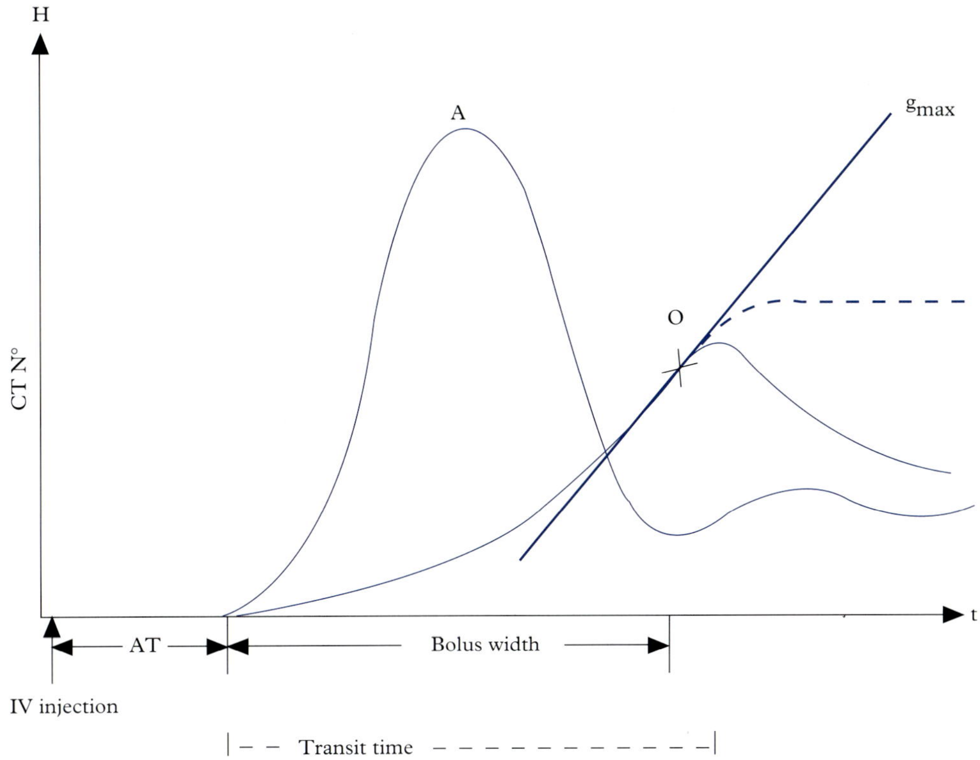

Figure 3.14
A CT N°–time curve indicating the approximate tissue/organ transit time. The peak is not reached so the Mullani–Gould method cannot be used. The peak gradient is reached in a shorter time and so the gradient method may be used (see Chapters 4 and 6). The mean transit time for the kidney is ~ 6 s.

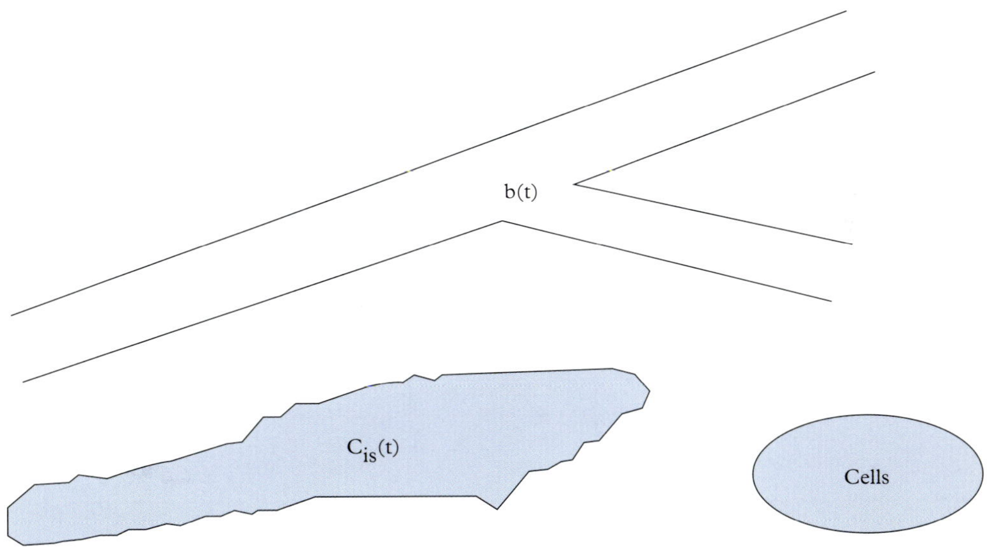

Figure 3.15
The compartments of (non-renal) tissue cellular, interstitial and vascular spaces. Contrast agents distribute themselves. Intracellular entry is negligible.

If ϕ_c is the proportionate cellular volume,

$$\phi_c + \phi_b + \phi_{is} = 1 \tag{6}$$

If we divide Equation (5) by $b(t)$,

$$\frac{c(t)}{b(t)} = \phi_{is}\frac{C_{is}(t)}{b(t)} + \phi_b \tag{7}$$

If $p(t)$ is the plasma concentration, $b(t) = (1 - \text{Hct})p(t)$ where Hct is the haematocrit. So

$$\frac{c(t)}{b(t)} = \phi_{\text{is}} \frac{C_{\text{is}}(t)}{(1 - \text{Hct})p(t)} + \phi_{\text{b}}$$

Now, since CT N° is proportional to contrast/iodine concentration, we may replace all the concentrations in the above equations by CT N°. $c(t)$ becomes the CT N° of a tissue region of interest, $b(t)$ the blood CT N°. $C_{\text{is}}(t)$ cannot, of course, be measured directly.

Such simple considerations allow a clearer understanding of CT enhancement in anatomical imaging studies to be achieved as well as forming the basis for functional studies. As regards the latter, we may see how some useful information may be obtained quite readily.

At early time, $C_{\text{is}}(t) \approx 0$ so

$$\frac{c(t)}{b(t)} \sim \phi_{\text{b}}$$

At later t, $C_{\text{is}}(t) \sim p(t)$ (equilibrium phase) so

$$\frac{c(t)}{b(t)} \sim \phi_{\text{b}} + \frac{\phi_{\text{is}}}{1 - \text{Hct}}$$

If a series of values of $c(t)$ and $b(t)$ are obtained from organ and arterial ROIs, respectively, a plot of the form shown in Figure 3.16 may be obtained. The curve deviates from its initial linearity because contrast exchange between blood and interstitium is a two-way process.

Thus ϕ_{b} and, with substitution of a value for haematocrit, ϕ_{is} may be obtained.

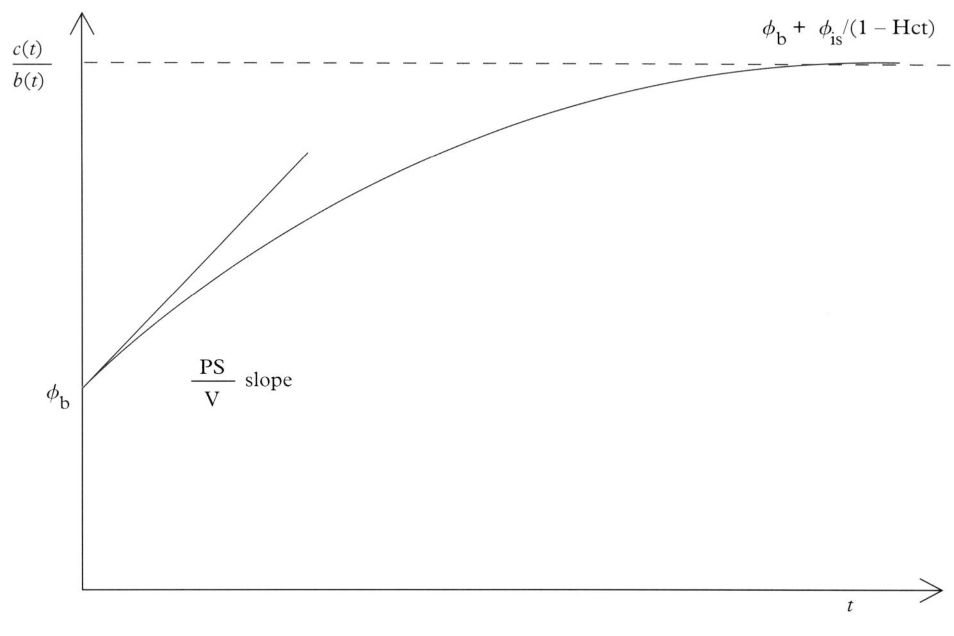

Figure 3.16
A diagrammatic plot of $c(t)/b(t)$ against time. The intercept is proportionate vascular volume, ϕ_{b}, the asymptote is $\phi_{\text{b}} + [\phi_{\text{is}}/(1 - \text{Hct})]$ and the initial slope is PS-product per unit volume.

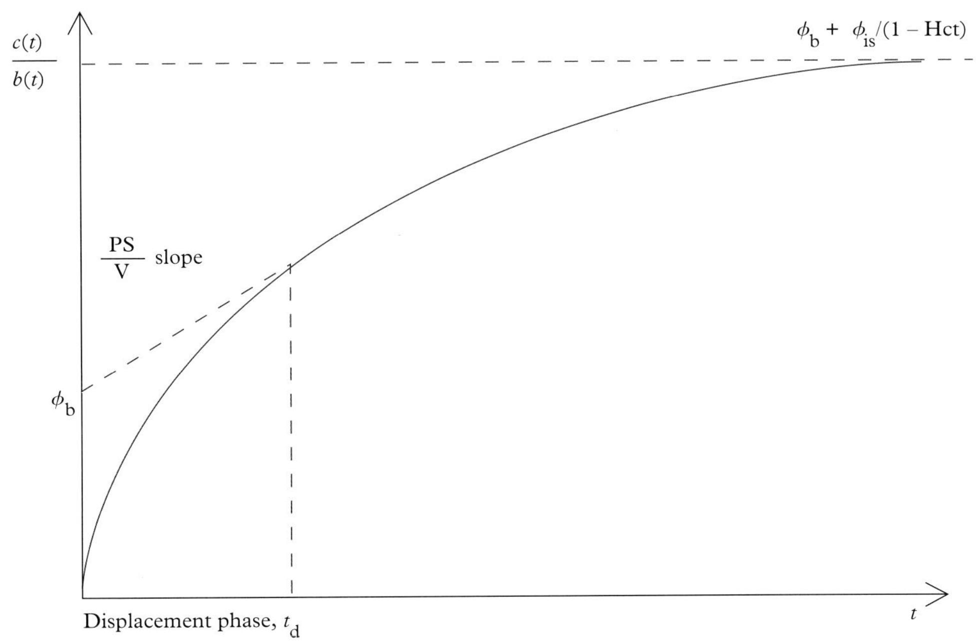

Figure 3.17
Figure 3.16 is not strictly accurate. There is an early phase of displacement of non-contrast filled blood of varying length t_d.

Using Equation 6, ϕ_c may then be calculated. The initial slope of the curve represents vascular permeability, PS-product per unit volume, in the ROI (see Chapter 10). These are all important parameters to the physiologist and anatomist and the differences between their values in normal and abnormal tissues may form the basis of an approach to tissue characterization studies.

In fact, the curves obtained are more like that illustrated in Figure 3.17. The early phase, of varying length in different tissues, represents the time during which displacement from the region of non-contrast containing blood occurs.

Chapters 5, 6 and 7 illustrate how making measurements in small regions of interest down to pixel level and colour-coding these values allows parametric maps to be generated to make clear perfusion variations and, in some cases, even to reveal a lesion not clearly seen using anatomical imaging. Such procedures may also be carried out on a variety of parameters other than perfusion such as regional PS-product, proportionate cellular volume, proportionate vascular volume and proportionate interstitial volume.

The above is an appropriate analysis for iodinated X-ray (or Gd-chelate magnetic resonance) contrast-enhancing agents which are ECF markers. A different mathematical approach may be taken if a 'blood-pool' agent is used and this is explored in Chapter 4. For the specific case of the normal brain, ECF agents may be considered to be 'blood-pool' agents because of the blood–brain barrier (BBB).

THE KIDNEY

The kidney is of special interest for a number of reasons and the assessment of its blood flow/perfusion and GFR are important aims. In other tissues, the contrast agent tracer becomes distributed, as we have discussed, between plasma and interstitium. In the kidney, the distribution is between plasma and proximal tubules (filtrate). This begins immediately at first-pass. The interstitium of the kidney is small in volume and, to all intents and purposes (see Chapter 8), communicates freely with the plasma because of the great permeability of renal blood vessels. PS-product is therefore replaced in the kidney by GFR and the plot of the kind illustrated in Figure 3.16 is analogous to the Patlak plot first developed in positron emission tomography (PET) studies and subsequently adopted for use in renal nuclear medicine studies [23, 26]. This subject will be developed in Chapters 4 and 8.

BOLUS ADMINISTRATION

It is a commonplace observation that even rapid, brief bolus injections on one side of the circulation produce broader tracer concentration–time curves on the other. Even a δ-function intravenous injection, that is a mathematically idealized one delivered in a zero time period, will still produce an arterial density–time curve of finite width and height, dictated partly by the cardiac output, partly by the central volume of blood in which dilution of tracer occurs and partly by the range of transit times found in the lungs. This is the so-called 'response function' and this subject is touched upon in Chapter 4 in the discussion of linear systems-based approaches and transit time. A detailed discussion of vascular bolus dynamics has been published elsewhere [25].

CAN THE TECHNIQUE AFFECT THE MEASUREMENTS?

This is a fundamental question which must always be asked in any experiment but is particularly apposite here. Contrast agents, as discussed above, have toxicities manifested specifically by effects on a variety of physiological parameters and so cannot automatically be assumed, for all their shared pharmacokinetics, to behave exactly like, say, TcDTPA. This potential difficulty will now be reviewed.

Cardiovascular effects

X-ray contrast agents have effects on smooth muscle, both directly and possibly by shear-induced endothelin-derived relaxant factor (EDRF) release, which cause vasodilatation and hypotension [6,18]. A reflex tachycardia partly mitigates this. On the heart itself there are negative inotropic effects on pump function and negative chronotropic effects [19,27]. These are, of course, greatest when the injection is intracoronary and are much reduced when it is into a peripheral vein.

Non-ionic monomeric and, even more so, non-ionic dimeric agents, are associated with much less-marked effects in these regards [3,9,14].

Renal effects

The cardiac effects and effects on peripheral vasculature will tend to engender a reduction of renal blood flow and, consequently, GFR. In addition, there are specific effects, partly mediated by osmolality, which reduce renal blood flow after an initial rise; vasopressin release, stimulated by hyperosmolar agents, also has the same effect [16,17].

All these factors together might be expected to have an effect on GFR [28,29]. However, the non-ionic monomers and dimers have much reduced effects in every regard and produce little or, in the case of the dimers, no vasopressin or renal osmotic effects [9].

It seems reasonable to suppose that the peripheral venous injection of a modest bolus (say 25 ml) of a non-ionic monomeric or dimeric X-ray contrast agent will have little effect on cardiac output, blood pressure, tissue perfusion or GFR. Perhaps the best evidence for this may be found in the measurements of perfusion in the kidney, discussed in Chapters 6 and 7 which are close to the 'gold standard' found by more invasive measurements [30].

In general terms, the non-ionic agents are to be preferred for the reason that they are associated with reduced patient movement, including respiratory movements, swallowing, coughing, etc. (see also Chapter 5).

SUMMARY

Contrast agents, initially designed as their name suggests, for the enhancement of image contrast and diagnostic content, may also be used as tracers in a manner akin to the use of radioactive tracers in nuclear medicine. A number of parameters of physiological and clinical interest may be measured on this basis using modern fast CT. In principle, such methods are applicable to MRI and US with their appropriate contrast agents, but the outstanding advantage of CT lies in the linear nature of the CT N°.

The non-ionic agents are particularly suitable for such procedures, in the modest doses required, and in the minimal effect they have on any of the parameters to be measured. The techniques and relevant mathematical analyses are enlarged upon in subsequent specialist sections of this book.

REFERENCES

1. Haschek, E. and Lindenthal, T.O. (1896) Ein Betrag zur praktischen Verwertung der Photographie nach Röntgen. *Wiener Klinische Wochenschrift*, **9**, 63–64.
2. Burrows, E.H. (1986) *Pioneers and Early Years. A History of British Radiology.* Alderney: Colophon Ltd.
3. Dawson, P. (1987) Radiological contrast agents in interventional radiology. *Journal of Interventional Radiology*, **2**, 51–58.

4. Dawson, P. and Blomley, M.J.K. (1994) Gadolinium chelate MR contrast agents. *Clinical Radiology*, **49**, 439–442.
5. Grainger, R.G. (1982) Intravascular contrast media — the past, the present and the future. *British Journal of Radiology*, **55**, 1–18.
6. Dawson, P., Grainger, R.G. and Pitfield, J. (1983) The new low osmolar contrast media. *Clinical Radiology*, **34**, 221–226.
7. Dawson, P. and Allison, D.J. (1989) Safer contrast agents. *British Journal of Hospital Medicine*, **42**, 406–407.
8. Dawson, P. and Howell, M.J. (1986) Pharmacology of the non-ionic dimers. *British Journal of Radiology*, **59**, 987–991.
9. Dawson, P., (1995) The non-ionic dimers. Some theoretical and clinical considerations. *European Radiology*, **5**, S103–S106.
10. Dawson, P., Turner, M.W., Bradshaw, A. and Westaby, S. (1983) Complement activation and generation of C_3A anaphylatoxin by radiological contrast agents. *British Journal of Radiology*, **56**, 447–448.
11. Assem, E.S.K., Bray, K. and Dawson, P. (1983) Release of histamine from human basophils by radiological contrast agents. *British Journal of Radiology*, **56**, 647–652.
12. Dawson, P. and Edgerton, D. (1983) Contrast media and enzyme inhibition. I. Cholinesterase. *British Journal of Radiology*, **56**, 653–656.
13. Dawson, P., Harrison, J.G. and Weisblatt, E. (1983) Effect of contrast media on red cell filtrability and morphology. *British Journal of Radiology*, **56**, 707–710.
14. Dawson, P. (1985) Chemotoxicity of contrast media and clinical adverse effects; a review. *Investigative Radiology*, **20**, 52–59.
15. Dawson, P., Hine, A.L. and Lui, D. (1985) Contrast agent osmolality and plasma volume changes. *Acta Radiologica*, **26**, 753–756.
16. Trewhella, M., Dawson, P., Rickards, D. and Forsling, M. (1987) Dehydration, ADH and the IVU. *British Journal of Radiology*, **60**, 445–447.
17. Dawson, P., Trewhella, M. and Forsling, M. (1990) Vasopressin release in response to intravenously injected contrast media. *British Journal of Radiology*, **63**, 97–100.
18. Pugh, N.D., Sissons, G.R. and Ruttley, M.S.T. (1993) The effect of iodixanol, a new non-ionic contrast agent on femoral blood flow in man. *Clinical Radiology*, **47**, 96–99.
19. Hayward, R. and Dawson, P. (1984) Contrast agents in angiocardiography. *British Heart Journal*, **52**, 361–368.
20. Dawson, P. (1991) Factors dictating iodinated contrast agent toxicity. In: *New Dimensions in Contrast Media*, (eds H. Katayama and R.C. Brasch) pp. 66–71. Amsterdam: Excerpta Medica.
21. Dawson, P. and Blomley, M.J.K. (1996) Contrast agents as extra-cellular fluid space markers: adaptation of the central volume theorem. *British Journal of Radiology*, **69**, 717–722.
22. Dawson, P. and Peters, A.M. (1996) Renal function and contrast elimination. *British Journal of Radiology*, **69**, 567–569.
23. Dawson, P. and Peters, A.M. (1993) Dynamic contrast bolus computed tomography for the assessment of renal function. *Investigative Radiology*, **28**, 1039–1042.
24. Dawson, P. (1996) Glomerular filtration rate determined using contrast clearance: should we all be doing it? *Current Opinion in Urology*, **6**, 75–77.
25. Blomley, M.J.K. and Dawson, P. (1997) Bolus dynamics: theoretical and experimental aspects. *British Journal of Radiology*, **70**, 351–359.
26. Blomley, M.J.K. and Dawson, P. (1996) The quantification of renal function with enhanced computerised tomography. *British Journal of Radiology*, **69**, 989–995.

27. Dawson, P. (1989) Cardiovascular effects of contrast agents. *American Journal of Cardiology*, **64**, 2E–9E.
28. Dawson, P. (1985) Contrast agent nephrotoxicity. An appraisal. *British Journal of Radiology*, **58**, 121–124.
29. Trewhella, M. and Dawson, P. (1990) Intravascular contrast agents and renal failure. *Clinical Radiology*, **41**, 373–375.
30. Blomley, M.J.K. and Dawson, P. (1993) Contrast bolus dynamic CT for the measurement of solid organ perfusion. *Investigative Radiology*, **28**, 572–577.

Chapter 4

THEORETICAL ASPECTS AND PHYSIOLOGICAL MODELS

M. Blomley and P. Dawson

This chapter will review the theoretical aspects of calculating physiological indices using intravascular injections of a contrast agent and computed tomography (CT). Before proceeding, it is necessary to deal with a fundamental assumption underpinning any such calculation — the assumption of linearity between the concentration of contrast agent and the change in CT number. Such a linear relationship is thought to exist on all commercial scanners but, ideally, should be confirmed prior to performing functional imaging studies. A calibration can be done (at least *in vitro*) easily using various dilutions of contrast agents and a phantom. In general, for each increase in average iodine concentration within a voxel by 1 mg/ml, CT number will increase by about 25 Hounsfield units (HU). The attenuation coefficient of iodine will vary from machine to machine, and with machine parameters, particularly tube kilo-voltage or kVp. Indeed, Hounsfield himself suggested that a dual-energy subtraction technique could be used to measure iodine concentration directly, although the technique has not found clinical applicability [1]. Such a linear relationship presumably exists for other high atomic number materials which could be used as X-ray contrast media, such as the gadolinium chelates, but should be confirmed if their use for functional imaging is contemplated. It should also be borne in mind that a linear relationship between CT number and contrast medium concentration *in vitro* is not a guarantee of linearity *in vivo*. Beam hardening, in particular, is a problem in some applications especially myocardial CT, where contrast medium within a chamber causes an under-estimate of myocardial attenuation and thus enhancement. In general, conditions which could give rise to non-linearity, such as very high concentrations of intravascular contrast, should be avoided. Nevertheless, in general and in most body and brain applications, non-linearity does not appear to be a major problem. This represents a major advantage of CT over the other cross-sectional imaging techniques of magnetic resonance and ultrasound (US). The interested reader is referred to a fuller discussion of these issues by Dean and Plewes [2].

A further assumption that needs to be made is that contrast medium does not perturb blood flow by, for example, producing vasodilation or vasoconstriction. Given that these assumptions can be made, it follows that the changes of CT number in a tissue or vascular region can be regarded as a form of time–concentration data. How can this be exploited to measure functional indices?

Two types of indices can be defined which, to some extent, reflect the two phases or volumes of distribution of the contrast agent: firstly, plasma and then extracellular fluid (ECF). Circulatory indices include fractional vascular volume, mean transit (MTT) time and, importantly, perfusion. Indices of the extracellular volume are more complex and essentially revolve around clearance or clearance per unit volume of ECF.

The most important of these indices is perfusion: flow per unit volume or mass of tissue. Since this represents blood flow normalized to the quantity of tissue supplied, it is clearly a very important measure of the microcirculation of a region. Historically, perfusion has usually been measured as flow per unit mass rather than volume which in part reflects the rather invasive techniques used to measure it (often *ex vivo* using animal models,) but it is in many ways more logical to normalize it with respect to volume and give it units of 'inverse time' or time^{-1}. Conversion between the two is not in any case difficult as most tissues have a specific gravity close to 1. Fractional vascular volume is an intuitively simple concept: a dimensionless number reflecting the proportion of tissue occupied by blood. Mean transit time (MTT) is rather more complex. It may be regarded as the response of an output vessel to an instantaneous unit impulse of contrast, but a full understanding requires a brief discussion of some aspects of linear-systems theory (see below). The three indices are intimately interrelated: indeed, perfusion is no more nor less than the ratio of fractional vascular volume to MTT.

Clearance is the ratio of the amount of contrast 'cleared' into a compartment (ECF or urine) to the blood or plasma concentration. Indices reflecting the extracellular component of contrast agent distribution are discussed further below, and in more detail in Chapter 8.

Several alternative mathematical approaches can be used for measurement of these indices. The choice is frequently a reflection of the type of information that is available for analysis. At the simplest level, a surprising amount of useful information can be extracted from a time–attenuation curve of a region of tissue without any information as to the input or output vascular concentrations. For example, there have been reports investigating the use of renal–time enhancement curves after a bolus of contrast in the kidney as an index of poor renal function or transplant rejection (Chapter 6). Such techniques, however, have not proved of great clinical value and probably have relatively little real potential as a true tool for physiological quantitation. For example, it is clear that a parenchymal time–attenuation curve after an intravenous injection of contrast will be influenced by cardiopulmonary transit as much as by the vasculature being studied. Considerably more information can be obtained if time–attenuation curves for feeding or draining vessels as well as tissue can be obtained in addition and used to normalize the data.

Two main mathematical approaches have been used for this type of work: simple compartmental analyses and linear systems-based approaches. These will be considered separately; compartmental analyses will be subdivided further in relation firstly to the determination of microcirculatory indices, and then to measurement of clearance and ECF transit.

COMPARTMENTAL ANALYSIS

Vascular measurements

This type of analysis may be seen as a 'black box' type of approach, where contrast medium is modelled as entering via an afferent artery, instantly distributing itself uniformly within the blood vessels and extracellular space of the tissue of interest, and then, after a short interval, starting to leave via an efferent vein. Although a simple model, this type of analysis is remarkably robust and can be used even if a significant amount of contrast diffuses into the extravascular space. A simple formulation of this model, variously referred to as the Sapirstein principle, the single-compartmental formulation and the Mullani–Gould relation, can be used to calculate perfusion.

Following a simple compartmental model, it calculates perfusion as the ratio of the maximal tissue attenuation increase to the area under the arterial time–density curve after correction for recirculation, ideally with a correction for venous outflow. This relationship may be seen simply as a restatement of the Law of Conservation of Mass. It is relatively easily derived from first principles as follows. At time t, let $a(t)$ be the arterial concentration of iodine, $v(t)$ the venous concentration and $c(t)$ the tissue concentration within a volume of tissue being examined. Write the volume of the voxel as V, and flow into the volume as F. Then by definition, the perfusion of the voxel is F/V. Consider the time interval $(t, t + \delta t)$. The amount of iodine arriving in this time is $F\delta t[a(t) - v(t)]$. This equals the change in the amount of iodine in the voxel, i.e. the change in $[Vc(t)]$.

Thus:

$$\delta[c(t)\ V] = V\ \delta[c(t)] = F\ \delta t[a(t) - v(t)]$$

Going to the limit and integrating with respect to t:

$$\frac{F}{V} = \frac{c(t)}{\int_0^t a(t)\mathrm{d}t - \int_0^t v(t)\mathrm{d}t} \qquad (1)$$

We thus have a way of measuring perfusion if we can simultaneously sample artery, vein and tissue iodine concentration. All that is necessary is to baseline-subtract the CT number of these regions, and to calculate the ratio of the increase in tissue CT number to the difference in areas under the arterial and venous time–attenuation curves (from the assumption of linearity discussed at the beginning of this chapter, changes in CT number are simply the increase in iodine density multiplied by a constant of proportionality, which is of course identical for numerator and denominator).

Unfortunately, few CT systems can simultaneously sample input, output and parenchymal areas reliably. This is only possible on electron-beam scanners with a multilevel capability at present but, as discussed in Chapter 6, such a machine has been used to measure renal cortical perfusion.

A much more typical situation, however, would be to have an arterial, but not venous, time–attenuation curve. A typical example would be in myocardial CT, where such curves can be constructed for the myocardium of the left ventricle and the left ventricular chamber (i.e. the input function). Equation (1) can then be adapted. If a reasonably short bolus of contrast has been given, we may reasonably assume that venous outflow is negligible for an appreciable time. Call this time t_{ven}. Then we may ignore $v(t)$ for $t < t_{ven}$. Perfusion may thus be calculated as:

$$\frac{F}{V} = \frac{c(t)}{\int_0^t a(t)\mathrm{d}t} (t < t_{ven}) \tag{2}$$

This ratio is best determined when numerator and denominator are a maximum, and error is reduced. Let t_{max} be the time of peak parenchymal enhancement. As long as $t_{max} < t_{ven}$ (and this is an important assumption, to which we shall return below),

$$\frac{F}{V} = \frac{c(t)|_{max}}{\int_0^{t_{max}} a(t)dt} \tag{3}$$

A refinement is to correct the vascular time–density curve for recirculation using a gamma-variate curve fit. In practice, vascular time–attenuation curves after a bolus of contrast have an initial maximum followed by a series of smaller peaks representing recirculation. The first-pass phase is easily modelled by a gamma-variate fit, that is, by a curve of the form

$$a(t) = k(t - t_0)^{\alpha} \mathrm{e}^{-(t - t_0)/\beta}$$

where $a(t)$ is the increase in vascular CT number over baseline, t is time, t_0 is the arrival time of contrast at the vascular region of interest (ROI) and k, α and β are constants which are parameters of the fit. The gamma-variate curve fit is a widely accepted method of extracting the initial (first-pass) phase from the time–concentration curve of a tracer [5].

If we perform a gamma-variate fit to the arterial time–density curve, to produce a fitted function $a^*(t)$, we may now calculate

$$\int_0^{\infty} a^*(t)\mathrm{d}t$$

as a measure of the area under the arterial curve if we had a tracer which did not undergo recirculation. The advantage of doing this is that we can adapt Equation (3) to be independent of t_{ven}, the time of venous outflow appearance. Perfusion is then calculated as

$$\frac{F}{V} = \frac{c(t)|_{max}}{\int_0^{\infty} a^*(t)dt} \tag{4}$$

Figure 4.1
Different techniques of calculating perfusion with a simple compartmental model.

(a) Simple compartmental model: the organ is considered to be in a 'black box' with time–concentration curve $c(t)$, supplied by an artery and vein with concentrations at time t of $a(t)$ and $v(t)$

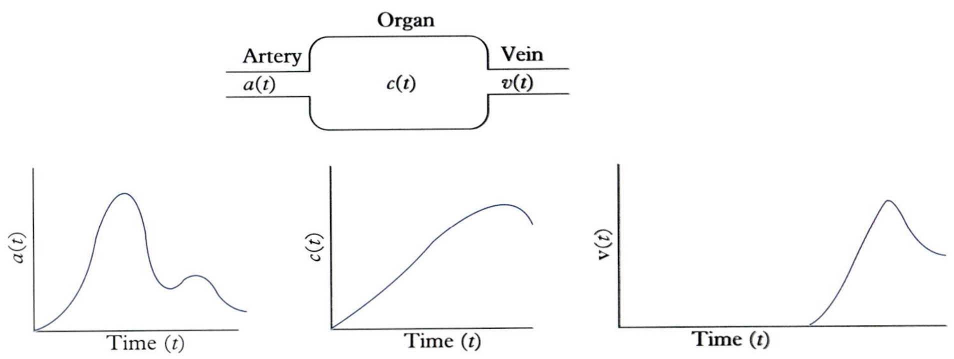

(b) If we integrate the arterial and venous–time concentration curves to time t, perfusion can then be calculated as:

$$\frac{c(t)}{\int_0^t a(t)\mathrm{d}t - \int_0^t v(t)\mathrm{d}t}$$

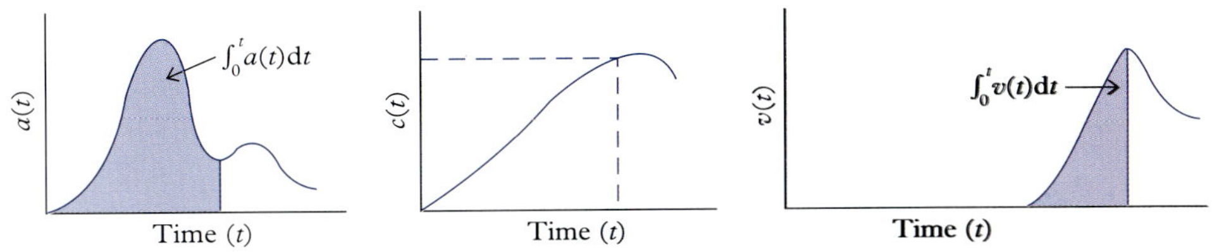

(c) If we correct the arterial time–density curve for recirculation $a^\star(t)$ and calculate the total area under the curve, perfusion can be calculated as the ratio of peak parenchymal density to this area:

$$\frac{c(t)|\max}{\int_0^\infty a^\star(t)\mathrm{d}t}$$

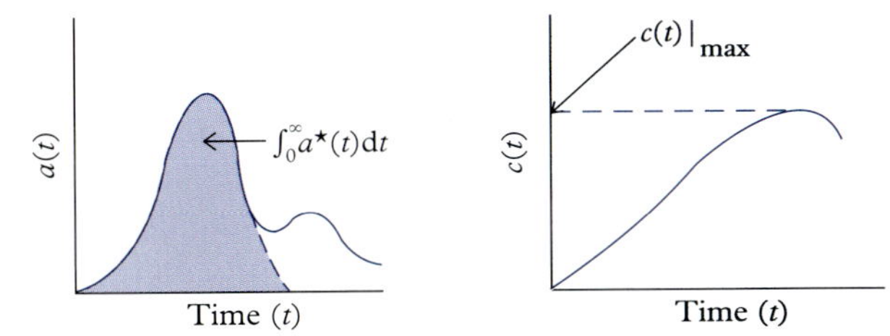

(d) Perfusion can also be calculated as the peak gradient of the tissue time–concentration curve, divided by the peak arterial concentration:

$$\frac{\left.\frac{\mathrm{d}c(t)}{\mathrm{d}t}\right|_{\max}}{a(t)|\max}$$

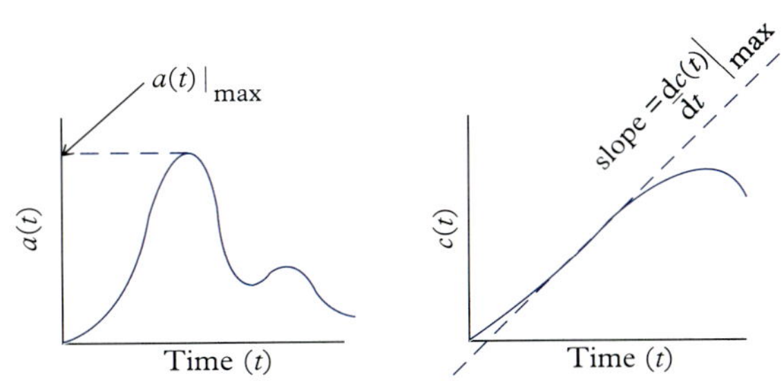

In other words, the ratio of the maximal tissue attenuation increase to the area under the arterial time–density curve after correction for recirculation.

This simple relationship, sometimes described as the Sapirstein or Mullani–Gould formulation [3,4], has given encouraging results in myocardial CT [6–11] (see Chapter 9) but unfortunately underestimates higher values of perfusion with intravenous injections because the assumption of 'no venous wash-out' is violated. For the algorithm to work, we require that the time to peak of the tissue time–density curve (i.e. the width of the input bolus) is longer than the minimum transit time of the system.

The same algorithm may be applied to abdominal and other applications by using the aorta as an 'input function'. Note that this implies that we make a further assumption — that there is no significant broadening or other perturbation of the time–attenuation curve between the aorta and the afferent arterioles. This should generally be the case, but would break down if there was a stenosis between the aorta and the relevant afferent arterioles. For example, renal cortical perfusion would be falsely underestimated if there were a renal artery stenosis.

Equations (1)–(3) may easily be rearranged and differentiated. If we do this, we obtain respectively:

Equation (5), derived from Equation (1):

$$\frac{F}{V} = \frac{\frac{\mathrm{d}}{\mathrm{d}t}[c(t)]}{a(t) - v(t)} \tag{5}$$

Equation (6), derived from Equation (2):

$$\frac{F}{V} = \frac{\frac{\mathrm{d}}{\mathrm{d}t}[c(t)]}{a(t)} (t < t_{\mathrm{ven}}) \tag{6}$$

Once again, error is minimized by taking the peak value of denominator and numerator. Let t^*_{max} be the time of the peak *gradient* of parenchymal enhancement, i.e. the peak up-slope of the tissue time–attenuation curve. As long as $t^*_{\mathrm{max}} < t_{\mathrm{ven}}$ we obtain:

Equation (7), derived from Equation (3)

$$\frac{F}{V} = \frac{\frac{\mathrm{d}}{\mathrm{d}t} c(t)|\mathrm{max}}{a(t_{\mathrm{max}})} \tag{7}$$

It is no longer necessary to perform a gamma-variate fit, as we did for Equation (4), although some data smoothing or curve fitting may be helpful and the gamma-fit is a helpful way of doing this.

Let us examine this relationship in more detail. If we assume there is minimal distortion of the vascular time–attenuation curve in passage from the artery we are measuring and the afferent arteriole (so that the maxima are identical), we may write:

$$\text{Perfusion} = \frac{\text{Peak gradient of the tissue time–attenuation curve}}{\text{Peak increase in arterial attenuation}}$$

This 'gradient relationship', widely used in this book, has certain powerful advantages over the Sapirstein/Mullani–Gould relationship. Notice that the tissue time–attenuation curve will reach its peak gradient (at t^*_{max}) well before its peak value (at t_{max}). Because we need only assume that no venous wash-out occurs before the time at which the tissue reaches its peak gradient t^*_{max}, not the later peak time t_{max}, the relationship is much less susceptible to an underestimate from venous wash-out. Another advantage is that it uses early time points (to define a peak gradient), which is often more practical when scanning on a single breath-hold. Its main disadvantage is that it is innately substantially more noise sensitive, as we are differentiating a dataset [11–14].

This gradient method is, incidentally, analogous to a previously described method of measuring blood flow using radionuclide angiography, which has been validated using microspheres. The problem of venous wash-out has been specifically addressed using the isotope method. Although relatively robust, large volume injections (using 50 ml given by hand) have been shown to produce errors in calculating blood flow when using the gradient method, and this should be borne in mind. Thus it reduces, but does not eliminate, the problem of wash-out error. In general, with all compartmental analyses, the smallest possible volume should be given as rapidly as possible [15–17].

These compartmental techniques can be extended to the dual blood supply of the liver as it is possible to define liver, spleno-portal and aortic vascular time–attenuation curves with single-level scanning. As discussed later in more detail (Chapter 6), one approach is to assume that no portal venous perfusion occurs before the time of peak splenic enhancement. Hepatic arterial perfusion can be determined using the gradient algorithm, with the aorta as input function and with the live time–attenuation curve only analysed prior to the time of peak splenic enhancement. Liver portal perfusion can then be analysed by dividing the late-phase up-slope of the liver time–attenuation curve by the peak increase in portal venous enhancement after correction for the arterial component [18].

A further index, fractional vascular volume, can be estimated using the ratio of the peak up-slopes or areas under the curve of the time–attenuation curves of an input vessel and the parenchyma [7]. Note, however, that this method assumes haematocrit is the same in large and small vessels. Unfortunately, tissue haematocrit is typically a fraction of its value in larger vessels (a point often not appreciated in the literature on this subject) and this approach should be used with caution.

Note also that cardiac output can be estimated from CT: it will be proportional to the ratio of the amount of contrast given to the area under a vascular (e.g. left ventricular) region of interest. This is discussed more fully in Chapter 9.

Diffusion outwith vessels

The simple 'black box' approach can be used to look at diffusion outside of the blood vessels. As described in Chapter 3, contrast agent pharmacokinetics can be modelled using a two-compartmental 'open' model, with rapid diffusion from the plasma to the ECF. In principle, it would be possible to use such a model fully and try to calculate rate constants for plasma–ECF exchange. Such an approach has recently become popular in some functional magnetic resonance imaging (MRI) applications, but has not been widely applied to CT. A simpler approach is the graphical Patlak analysis, named after its inventor, and originally developed for positron emission tomography (PET) [19].

If we administer a bolus of contrast medium and scan sequentially at one level through tissues and an input vessel after a short delay to allow mixing of the contrast in the plasma, we can construct time–attenuation curves for renal and aortic ROI, in a manner not dissimilar to that used for the measurement of perfusion.

Suppose that at time t, the blood-iodine concentration is uniformly distributed between all blood vessels with concentration $b(t)$ and in a volume of kidney the average concentration is $c(t)$. Let $Q(t)$ represent the total amount of iodine in a volume of size V, so $Q(t) = Vc(t)$. This can be considered to represent iodine in the tissue blood volume, $Q_b(t)$ and in the tissue ECF, $Q_{\mathrm{is}}(t)$. Let the blood volume within V be V_b. Clearly, by definition

$$Q(t) = Q_b(t) + Q_{\mathrm{is}}(t)$$

Now assume one-way transfer from the plasma to the ECF and that haematocrit is constant so that blood and plasma iodine concentrations are in proportion. Then d/dt $[Q_{\mathrm{is}}(t)] = \alpha b(t)$ where α is a constant of proportionality and $b(t)$ is the average blood concentration, and so

$$Q_{\mathrm{is}}(t) = \alpha \int b(t)\mathrm{d}t$$

Note that α is the rate of elimination of contrast divided by blood concentration which is, by definition, blood clearance.

Dividing by V

$$c(t) = \frac{C(t)}{V} = \frac{Q_b(t)}{V} + \frac{Q_{\mathrm{is}}(t)}{V}$$

Hence

$$\frac{c(t)}{b(t)} = \frac{Q_b(t)}{Vb(t)} + \frac{\alpha}{V}\frac{\int b(t)\mathrm{d}t}{b(t)}$$

Now if $Q_b(t) = V_B b(t)$. Then

$$\frac{c(t)}{b(t)} = \frac{V_{\mathrm{B}}}{V} + \frac{\alpha}{V}\frac{\int b(t)\mathrm{d}t}{b(t)}$$

But V_{B}/V is the fractional vascular volume (ϕ_B) of the tissue. We conclude

$$\frac{c(t)}{b(t)} = \phi_B + \frac{\alpha}{V}\frac{\int b(t)\mathrm{d}t}{b(t)}$$

The value of this to our CT data is not immediately obvious. However, suppose we plot on one axis the value $\int b^*(t)\mathrm{d}t/b(t)$ where $b^*(t)$ is the baseline-subtracted aortic CT number. This index has units of time and is sometimes called 'normalized time'. Suppose we also plot on another axis the ratio $c^*(t)/b^*(t)$ where $c^*(t)$ is the baseline-subtracted CT number of a renal ROI. The result should be a straight line, the y-axis intercept of which will estimate ϕ_B, and the

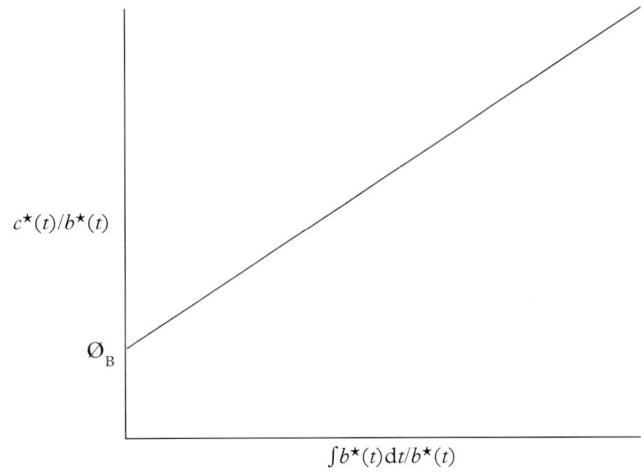

Figure 4.2
A Patlak plot. $b^\star(t)$ is the baseline subtracted aortic CT number, and $c^\star(t)$ the corresponding parenchymal CT number. The intercept on the y-axis will estimate fractional vascular volume (ϕ_B), and the gradient clearance per unit volume.

gradient of which will measure blood clearance per unit volume (Figure 4.2). Although there are limitations to this approach, and it is probably not correct to assume haematocrit is constant in different vascular beds, the technique has proved encouraging and its use is explored in Chapter 8.

Another aspect of the compartmental model applied to contrast agents is that in the late phase of distribution, excretion will become monoexponential with a rate constant which estimates glomerular filtration rate per unit volume. This is again discussed in Chapter 8.

LINEAR SYSTEMS-BASED APPROACHES AND TRANSIT TIME

Another approach to modelling blood flow through a tissue is to use the theory of time-invariant linear systems. This theory provides a fuller, but more complex, technique of analysis. The properties of such systems have been studied extensively in the physical sciences and by mathematicians, and this chapter will not attempt to discuss them in detail [20]. Whereas in compartmental models, flow through a system was seen as flow through a chain of compartments, within each of which there is complete and instant mixing, linear systems theory allows for a range of responses and transit times. Specifically, an instantaneous unit injection into an input vessel (a so-called 'delta' function) is modelled as producing a complex, possibly prolonged, response over time in an output vessel. This response function represents the distribution of transit times within the tissue. In principle, we could come close to measuring this if we could give a very small fast injection directly into a feeding artery to a tissue of interest, but this is not really practical for most CT applications.

The response functions within our systems can be analysed if they have certain basic properties:

- time-invariance (the behaviour after a given injection is constant);
- superposition (if an input x_1 causes an output y_1 and input x_2 causes an output

y_2, then a system is linear if, and only if, an input $x_1 + x_2$ causes an output $y_1 + y_2$;

- homogeneity (if an input x causes an output y then an input ax causes an output ay where a is a constant).

We can characterize the signal going past a point (say, the mid-aorta or left ventricle) by a quantity referred to as the 'mean transit time' (MTT), the 'centroid' or 'weighted first moment of the time–signal curve'. Suppose, a bolus intravenous injection is given and we are interested in the renal circulation. Write renal arterial concentration at time t as $a(t)$. The mean transit time of the renal artery is the ratio:

$$\mathrm{MTT_a} = \frac{\int_0^\infty t a(t)\,\mathrm{d}t}{\int_0^\infty a(t)\,\mathrm{d}t}$$

Likewise, we can define the MTT of the renal vein, $v(t)$:

$$\mathrm{MTT_v} = \frac{\int_0^\infty t v(t)\,\mathrm{d}t}{\int_0^\infty v(t)\,\mathrm{d}t}$$

If we ignore recirculation (and we can do this through the use of a gamma-variate fit) and if we assume our contrast agent remains intravascular, then the system mean transit time ($\mathrm{MTT_s}$), that is the mean transit time in the renal vein to a 'delta function' injection, can be calculated as the difference of these two:

$$\mathrm{MTT_s} = \mathrm{MTT_v} - \mathrm{MTT_a} = \frac{\int_0^\infty t v(t)\,\mathrm{d}t}{\int_0^\infty v(t)\,\mathrm{d}t} - \frac{\int_0^\infty t a(t)\,\mathrm{d}t}{\int_0^\infty a(t)\,\mathrm{d}t}$$

This $\mathrm{MTT_s}$ encapsulates many of the properties of the microcirculation within a tissue. For example, it might be short if multiple abnormal arteriovenous shunts existed within a tumour bed, or prolonged in a obliterative microangiopathy. Furthermore, it is possible to show that

$$\text{Perfusion} = \frac{\text{fvv}}{\mathrm{MTT_s}}$$

or perfusion is the ratio of fractional vascular volume to $\mathrm{MTT_s}$ [21]. This, the 'central volume theorem', provides an alternative approach to the measurement of perfusion. Either we can attempt to measure fractional vascular volume as described above, or we can simply use the reciprocal of MTT as a yardstick for changes in perfusion. Using this latter approach, Jaschke *et al.* have obtained an impressive correlation with perfusion measured using renal ultrafast CT [22].

Unfortunately it is not applicable to many CT applications as once again we need to sample both output and input vessels.

Note, importantly, that we need to assume our contrast agent remains intravascular for this type of analysis. As Chapter 3 has shown, this is difficult to do in many CT applications as contrast extravasates rapidly into the tissue extravascular spaces. It is not unreasonable to apply this type of analysis to the brain, however, as the blood–brain barrier is generally fairly impermeable. On theoretical grounds, non-ionic agents and particularly dimeric agents offer theoretical advantages here as they should be better retained within the vascular space.

Once again, we have so far only developed an analysis suitable for studying enhancement where the input, output and parenchymal curves can be characterized. Can we measure $\mathrm{MTT_s}$ from the parenchymal and input curves? The answer is probably not in a rigorous sense, but we can attempt to estimate it. In order to do this, we need to make certain assumptions about the distribution of transit times within a system. In careful work, Gobbel *et al.* describe the theoretical aspects of this type of analysis and demonstrate how it can be used to measure regional blood flow within the dog brain using time–attenuation data from different areas and an arterial input vessel seen on the scan plane. They calculate perfusion using the relationship,

$$\text{Perfusion} = n\frac{\int_0^\infty c(t)\mathrm{d}t}{\int_0^\infty a(t)\mathrm{d}t}(\mathrm{MTT_s} - \mathrm{MTT_a})$$

where n is the factor

$$n = \frac{(1 - \mathrm{Hct_{art}})(1 + k^2)}{2(1 - j\mathrm{Hct_{art}})(1 - m)}$$

Here Hct_{art} is the arterial haematocrit, j is a factor estimating the difference between tissue and large vessel haematocrit, k is the normalized standard deviation of transit times through the tissue, and m is a factor allowing for the time lag between the vessel studied and the tissue ROI [23,24].

CONCLUSION

There are, clearly, from the above discussion, considerable problems in applying linear systems-based approaches to the measurement of perfusion and flow in CT although they may have some applications in the brain. At present, the most promising techniques appear to be the use of simple compartmental analyses, and the gradient technique, as described above, which is simple and relatively robust, seems the best all-round method of measuring perfusion.

REFERENCES

1. Hounsfield, G.N. (1973) Computerized transverse axial scanning (tomography): I. Description of systems. *British Journal of Radiology*, **46**, 1016–1022.
2. Dean, P.B. and Plewes, D.B. (1984) Contrast media in computed tomography. In: *Radiocontrast Agents* (ed. M. Sovak). Berlin: Springer Verlag.
3. Sapirstein, L.A. (1958) Regional blood flow by fractional distribution of indicators. *American Journal of Physiology*, **193**, 161–168.
4. Mullani, N. and Gould, R.J. (1983) First pass measurement of regional blood flow using external detectors. *Journal of Nuclear Medicine*, **24**, 577–581.
5. Thompson, H.K., Starmer, C.F., Whalen, R.E. and McIntosh, H.D. (1963) Indicator transit time considered as a gamma variate. *Circulation Research*, **14**, 502–515.
6. Gould, R.G., Lipton, M.J., MacNamara, M.T., Sievers, R.E., Koshold, S. and Higgins, C.B. (1988) Measurement of regional myocardial blood flow in dogs by ultrafast CT. *Investigative Radiology*, **23**(5), 348–353.
7. Rumberger, J.A., Feiring, A.J., Lipton, M.J., Higgins, C.B., Ell, S.R. and Marcus, M.L. (1987) Use of ultrafast computed tomography to quantitate myocardial perfusion; a preliminary report. *Journal of the American College of Cardiology*, **9**, 59–69.
8. Wolfkiel, C.J., Ferguson, J.L., Chomka, E.V., Law, W.R., Labin, I.N., Tenzer, M.L., Booker, M. and Brundage, B.H. (1987) Measurement of myocardial blood flow by ultrafast computed tomography. *Circulation*, **76**, 1262–1273.
9. Rumberger, J.A. and Bell, M.R. (1992) Measurement of myocardial perfusion and cardiac output using intravenous injection methods by ultrafast (cine) computed tomography. *Investigative Radiology*, **27**(Suppl 2), S40–S46.
10. Gould, R.G. (1992) Perfusion quantification by ultrafast computed tomography. *Investigative Radiology*, **27**(Suppl 2), S18–S21.
11. Wolfkiel, C.J. and Brundage, B.H. (1991) Measurement of myocardial blood flow by UFCT: towards clinical applicability. *International Journal of Cardiac Imaging*, **7**, 89–101.
12. Miles, K.A. (1991) Measurement of tissue perfusion by dynamic computed tomography. *British Journal of Radiology*, **64**, 409–412.
13. Miles, K.A., Hayball, M.P. and Dixon, A.K. (1994) Functional imaging of changes in human intrarenal perfusion using quantitative dynamic computed tomography. *Investigative Radiology*, **29**, 911–914.
14. Blomley, M.J.K., Kormano, M, Coulden R. *et al.* (1994) Renal perfusion quantified with contrast enhanced CT. *Investigative Radiology*, **29(2)**, S232–33.
15. Peters, A.M., Gunasekera, R., Henderson, B.L., Brown, J., Lavender, J.P., De Souza, M., Ash, J.M. and Gilday, D.L. (1987) Non-invasive measurement of blood flow and extraction fraction. *Nuclear Medicine Communications*, **8**, 823–837.
16. Peters, A.M., Brown, J., Hartnell, G.G., Myers, M., Haskell, M.J. and Lavender, J.P. (1987) Non-invasive measurement of renal blood flow with Tc-99m DTPA: a comparison with microspheres. *Cardiovascular Research*, **21**, 830–834.
17. Bell, S.D. and Peters, A.M. (1991) Measurement of blood flow from first pass radionuclide angiography: influence of bolus volume. *European Journal of Nuclear Medicine*, **18**, 885–888.
18. Blomley, M.J.K., Coulden R., Dawson, P., Kormano, M., Donlan, P., Bufkin, C. and Lipton M.J. (1995) Liver perfusion studies with dynamic computed tomography. *Journal of Computer Assisted Tomography*, **19(3)**, 424–433.

19. Patlak C.S., Blasberg R.G., Fernstmacher J.D. (1983) Graphical evaluation of blood to brain transfer constants from multiple time uptake data. *Journal of Cerebral Flow and Metabolism*, **3**, 1–7.
20. Blomley, M.J.K. and Dawson, P. (1996) The quantification of renal function with enhanced computed tomography. *British Journal of Radiology*, **69**, 989–995.
21. Maier, P. and Zierler, K.L. (1954) On the theory of indicator dilution method for the measurement of blood flow and volume. *Journal of Applied Physiology*, **4**, 308–314.
22. Jaschke, W.R., Gould, R.G., Cogan, M.G., Sievers, R. and Lipton, M.J. (1987) Cine-CT measurement of cortical renal blood flow. *Journal of Computer Assisted Tomography*, **11**(5), 779–784.
23. Gobbel, G.T., Cann, C.E. and Fike, J.R. (1991) Measurement of regional cerebral blood flow using ultrafast computed tomography: theoretical aspects. *Stroke*, **22**, 768–771.
24. Gobbel, G.T., Cann, C.E., Iwamato, H.S. and Fike, J.R. (1991) Measurement of regional cerebral blood flow in the dog using ultrafast computed tomography; experimental validation. *Stroke*, **22**(6), 772–779.

Chapter 5

CT PERFUSION TECHNIQUES

K. Miles and M. Blomley

The measurement of perfusion with computed tomography (CT) requires accurate determination of parenchymal and vascular time–attenuation curves after an injection of contrast medium. At least one baseline-unenhanced image is required (so as to define baseline attenuation values) followed by a rapid sequence of data acquisitions without table movement after an intravenous bolus of contrast medium. The sequence should comprise enough images to allow characterization of the relevant portions of the tissue and vessel time–attenuation curves with respect to the algorithm being used to determine perfusion. It is, of course, vital that misregistration of consecutive images due to respiration or other movement is minimized. This type of imaging protocol is often referred to as a *single-location dynamic sequence*.

In practical terms, sufficient scans are required firstly to enable an accurate curve-fitting procedure, such as a gamma-variate or cubic spline function, to be performed on the time–attenuation data from the input vessel (or left ventricle in the case of cardiac studies) and secondly to characterize the wash-in phase of the tissue time–attenuation curve. For some perfusion algorithms, time–attenuation data from an output vessel or inclusion of the tissue wash-out phase may also be helpful. The total number of images and the sampling frequency has to be a compromise between improved accuracy with high temporal resolution on the one hand and increased radiation dose to the patient and machine limitations on the other. The exact technique used may, therefore, vary between CT systems and depend upon the nature of the contrast input injection and the tissue under investigation. The CT system requirements for performing perfusion studies are outlined in Table 5.1. In many cases, particularly with intravenous injections, a conventional CT system is adequate. However, if a central venous injection is being used to study pulmonary or myocardial perfusion, the rapid subsecond scanning capabilities of electron-beam systems would be necessary. Unless otherwise stated, this chapter will concentrate on the technique for studying perfusion in the solid organs using an intravenous injection of contrast medium.

Two recent developments in CT system design may have benefits for perfusion imaging. Systems that simultaneously acquire two slices will allow a greater volume of tissue to be studied with one contrast medium injection. Also, it may be possible to correct for excessive respiratory motion by selecting the most appropriate images from either set of images. The second development is rapid reconstruction times combined with a continually rotating gantry, allowing

Essential
Single location sequence capability
Data acquisitions at least every 3 s
Tube cooling characteristics allowing ten acquisitions within 40 s
Attenuation values can be determined from identical ROIs from each image
Desirable
Data acquisition times of 1 s or less
Variable interscan delay
Dynamic evaluation software (including gamma-variate curve fitting)
Reconstructed-image data transferable to separate workstation

Table 5.1
CT system requirements for perfusion CT

'real-time' imaging. This system could allow the necessary data sequence to be commenced at the moment contrast medium arrives in the aorta, either visually or automatically using a predetermined threshold aortic attenuation value. This facility would be particularly useful in patients with prolonged circulation time, such as the elderly, or in patients with impaired cardiac function, and could obviate dye detection techniques (e.g. indocyanine green) sometimes used to determine circulation times prior to dynamic CT scanning (see Chapter 9).

CHOICE OF SLICE LEVEL

The slice chosen for study is selected from an initial conventional incremental sequence of images. The single-location perfusion sequence will be performed either with breath-holding (if feasible) or with the patient breathing quietly, and thus this initial series of images should be performed with identical breathing instructions so that the slice chosen will correspond as closely as possible with the slice for the perfusion study. As well as including the organ or lesion under study, it is important to identify a suitable blood vessel (or cardiac chamber) for construction of a vascular reference region of interest (ROI). Ideally, the vessel will be perpendicular to the slice and large enough to create a ROI of sufficient size to avoid partial volume effects. The vessel should also remain stationary during the study. Within the chest and upper abdomen, the aorta is usually the most appropriate choice. In the absence of a clearly identifiable large vessel, such as in the brain, the vascular ROI can be chosen after the perfusion image sequence, at the analysis stage (see below).

For separate analysis of hepatic arterial and portal perfusion, an additional reference ROI is required. If using the *indirect* or *splenic fit methods*, a splenic ROI is required. When using the *direct method* (see Chapter 6) for measuring portal perfusion, a portal or splenic vein ROI is also required. Depending on the analysis method used, either the time to peak splenic enhancement is used to separate hepatic arterial and portal venous phases or the splenic time–attenuation

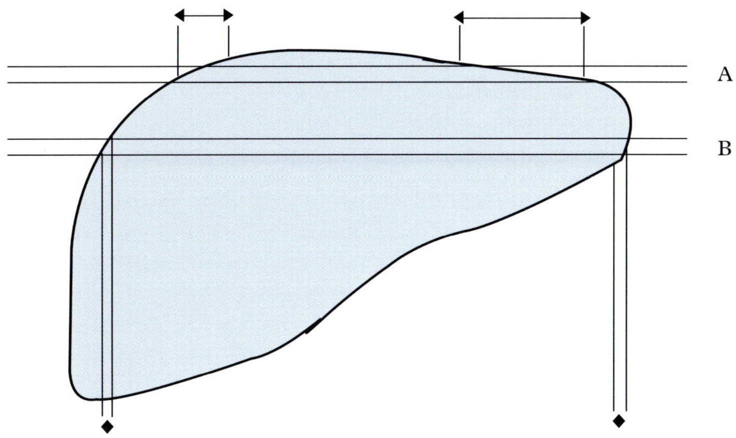

Figure 5.1
Slice A, close to the top of the liver, suffers much greater misregistration artefact (due to respiratory movement) than does slice B in the mid-portion of the liver.

curve provides a model for the hepatic arterial enhancement (see Chapter 6). If there has been a splenectomy, then the time to peak enhancement from the time–attenuation curve of another organ, such as renal cortex or pancreas, can be used as an alternative (for the *indirect portal method*).

Wherever possible, slice locations should be chosen to minimize motion artefact resulting from slight differences in the position of an organ between individual images from the sequence. Slices close to the cranial or caudal limits of an organ are particularly prone to motion artefact as small respiratory movements will be exaggerated (Figure 5.1). Similarly, when assessing hepatic perfusion in the absence of a focal lesion, for example in evaluating suspected diffuse liver disease, it is best to avoid slice locations close to the diaphragm. Cardiac motion will also create movement artefacts for chest studies (except when using electron-beam systems).

DATA ACQUISITION PROTOCOLS

As perfusion is calculated from changes in attenuation following contrast medium, a baseline unenhanced image is necessary so that attenuation values from this image can subsequently be subtracted from those derived from enhanced images. This baseline image is best defined as part of the single-location sequence rather than as a previously obtained image at the same level so as to minimize any differences in position of the patient. (This is also a prerequisite for some dynamic evaluation software packages). The start of this first acquisition can be conveniently used as a signal for the commencement of the contrast medium injection. If the CT system will allow, it is also useful to program a delay of 7–10 s between the baseline image and the first postcontrast image.

The frequency of data acquisitions thereafter is a compromise between improving the quality of data with more frequent acquisitions and minimizing the radiation burden to the patient. A variable interscan delay is of advantage as this enables frequent acquisitions to be acquired early in the sequence when contrast medium concentration is changing rapidly, particularly in the vascular system. Images during this phase should be performed sufficiently frequently to avoid underestimation of peak vascular enhancement. Such errors become less likely the closer the temporal spacing of the images and, although ideally acquisitions every second (or even less) are desirable in this phase, from a pragmatic point of view, it is sufficient simply to aim to obtain several data points during the wash-in phase of vascular enhancement. To achieve this, scans early in the sequence should be performed no more than 3 s apart if using a 50 ml bolus of contrast medium (for smaller volumes, a more rapid sequence may be required).

Acquisitions can then be performed less frequently towards the end of the sequence when tissue concentrations are changing slowly. If data acquisitions are too infrequent, the maximal rate of tissue enhancement and hence the measured perfusion will be underestimated. The size of this error depends on the perfusion of the tissue concerned, but will be greater for highly perfused organs such as the renal cortex.

When using a maximum slope or gradient method of analysis (see Chapter 4), a complete sequence lasting for 30 s from the onset of injection is sufficient for most applications. For the Mullani–Gould analysis method, sequences should be 10 s longer. For the liver, a sequence lasting at least 40–45 s is required to include the portal venous phase of enhancement. A longer protocol is also appropriate for the spleen as the splenic matrix may enhance significantly later than lymphatic cords. It may be useful to perform a liver protocol whenever the liver is included on the slice studied, even if another organ is the organ of interest, as unsuspected liver disease may be discovered. Example protocols are given in Figure 5.2 and individual images from a typical single-location series for cerebral perfusion are shown in Figure 5.3. A slice thickness of 10 mm reduces photon noise ensuring the final perfusion images are of high spatial resolution. Noise is also reduced by selecting a 'soft-tissue' reconstruction algorithm which uses a back-projection filter with a lower cut-off frequency.

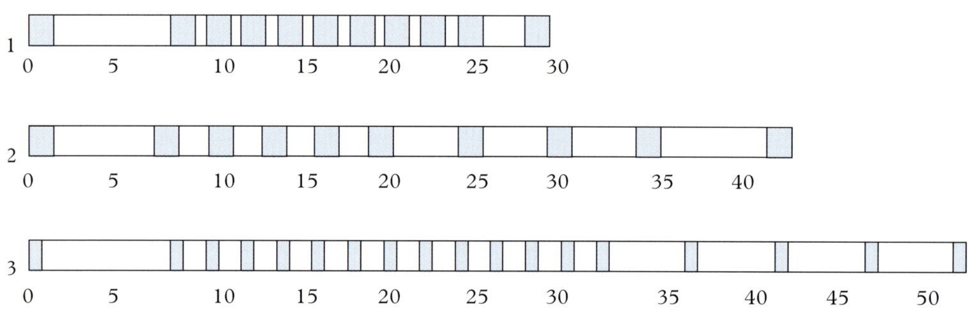

Figure 5.2
Time lines depicting example dynamic sequences for perfusion CT (times in seconds).
1. General perfusion protocol (gradient method) that allows for a breath-hold technique using a conventional CT system capable of 1 s scan times.
2. Liver perfusion protocol (quiet respiration) for a conventional CT system using a 1 s scan time.
3. General perfusion protocol for electron beam CT system using a 0.4 s scan time.

CONTRAST MEDIUM INJECTION

Non-ionic contrast media should be used for perfusion studies on account of the lower incidence of heat and flushing experienced by the patient as compared with ionic media. Such symptoms tend to increase movement of the patient,

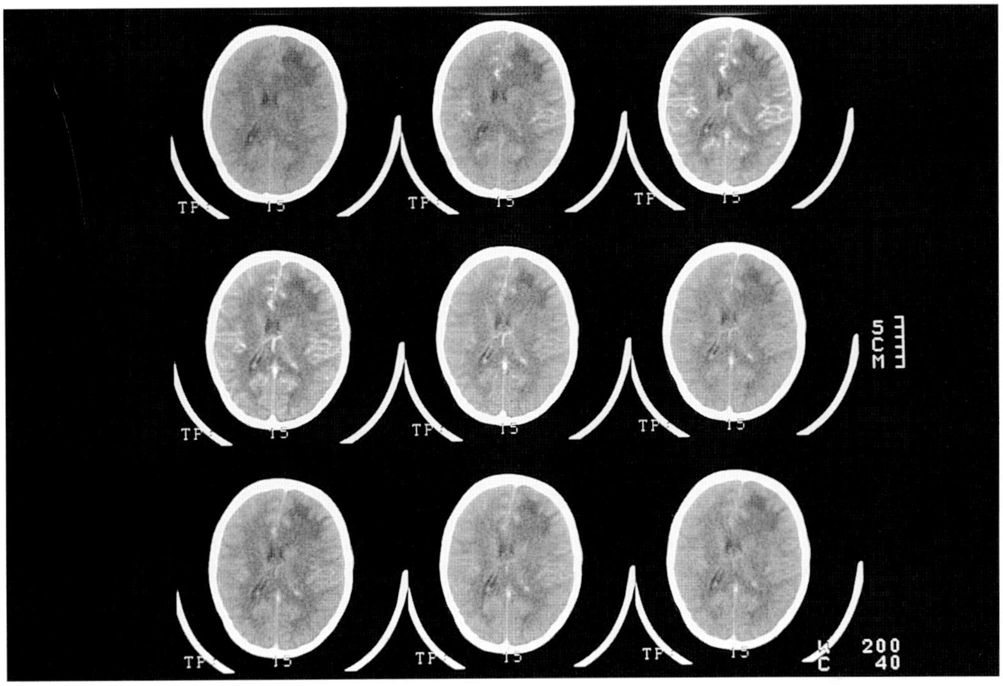

Figure 5.3
A series of nine images from a single-location sequence for measurement of cerebral perfusion using the gradient method of analysis.

particularly respiratory motion, and produce artefacts on subsequent perfusion images or errors in ROI perfusion calculations and thus should be kept to a minimum. Even when using non-ionic contrast media, the injection of contrast medium will usually induce in the patient a sensation of heat or flushing. If not forewarned of this effect, the patient will tend to respond by taking a deep inspiration, thereby producing significant respiratory motion artefacts. It is important to carefully instruct the patient before the study that he will experience a feeling of heat and that he should resist the temptation to take a deep breath but simply breath quietly throughout.

The lower osmolality of non-ionic agents is also associated with smaller negatively inotropic and chronotropic effects, particularly with intravenous injection, which should, in turn, result in a better aortic bolus. The vasodilatation (or vasoconstriction in the case of the kidney) produced by contrast media is unlikely to produce significant errors in perfusion measurements as the effect will be small within the first-pass. Nevertheless, the potential for such errors can be minimized by the use of non-ionic agents which are less likely to disturb the circulation of the organ under study. Low osmolar agents are also better retained within the vascular system which may be important if a linear system transit-time analysis is used (see Chapter 4).

As a rapid bolus is required, low viscosity is an advantage, especially if a hand injection is used. However, this should not be achieved by using a lower iodine concentration. Diluting the contrast medium will either increase the injected volume and result in poorer bolus geometry, or reduce the total iodine dose which will produce less tissue enhancement and a poorer signal-to-noise ratio. Warming the contrast medium to 30–37°C will usefully reduce the viscosity. Even with warm contrast medium, a 19-gauge or larger cannula or 'butterfly' needle is usually required to enable a sufficiently rapid injection.

When deciding upon the volume of contrast medium to be injected, there are conflicting priorities to consider. Clearly, for a given concentration, the greater the volume of contrast medium, the better will be the signal-to-noise ratio of the subsequent study. However, with larger volumes, it is harder to achieve a sufficiently narrow bolus shape within the aorta to satisfy the assumptions of the analysis algorithm, particularly if using the Mullani–Gould analysis without a correction for venous outflow (see Chapter 4). Furthermore, increasing the injection rate above a certain level (about 8–10 ml/s) does not produce further improvements in the bolus geometry due to mechanical buffering within the lung. In practice, volumes of 25–50 ml are usually satisfactory for intravenous injections in adult patients. Within that range, the exact volume is not critical, as the algorithms used for calculating perfusion are not dependent upon amount of contrast medium injected and the emphasis should be on duration rather than volume of injection. However, the *optimum* volume and duration of injection will vary with different target tissues. For organs that have relatively low perfusion and slower vascular transit (e.g. liver, brain, pancreas) a greater volume is desirable to increase the signal-to-noise ratio and 40–50 ml over 7 s or less (achievable with hand injection if required) produces results close to expected perfusion values for most organs when using the gradient method of analysis. For tissues such as renal cortex, that have high perfusion and more rapid vascular transit, a shorter injection of smaller volume may be more appropriate. For instance, 25 ml intravenous volumes have been used for studies of renal cortical perfusion with good results.

It is not necessary to standardize the rate of injection for all patients as this will not ensure consistency in bolus geometry between individuals. This is because other confounding factors, such as central blood volume and cardiac output, will have a significant influence on the resultant aortic bolus shape.

A practical approach, especially when using hand injections, is to use two data acquisitions as signals for starting and stopping the injection. The injection is begun as the first acquisition commences. The commencement of a second acquisition programmed 7 s after the baseline image provides the signal for terminating the injection no matter how much contrast medium has been administered.

DATA ANALYSIS

A cine display of the images from the single location dynamic sequence is an important quality-control procedure to evaluate the degree of movement of the patient, particularly if the acquisition protocol has allowed quiet respiration. Movement errors are also frequently apparent on visual inspection of time–attenuation data from a tissue ROI. Any images in which there has been a lot of movement should be excluded from analysis. If movement of the patient during the imaging sequence causes pixels of low attenuation adjacent to an organ (e.g. perinephric fat) to be replaced by contrast-enhanced tissue, a sudden decrease in attenuation will result thereby creating a falsely low-perfusion value for that pixel. Alternatively, high-attenuation material, such as bone, moving into a pixel during the sequence, will also create a spuriously high-perfusion value. Motion artefacts are most apparent on functional images of perfusion and, if severe, can render the perfusion images of no value. However, ROI data can often be salvaged from such studies as long as the ROI remains within the organ throughout the sequence.

A thresholding procedure enables movement artefacts to be minimized by eliminating from the analysis pixels containing material of very high or very low attenuation, such as bone, fat or air, that are prone to causing movement artefacts. Suitable thresholds are 0 HU to 400 HU with pixels of initial attenuation values outside these limits being excluded.

REGION OF INTEREST ANALYSIS

A quick and simple method of analysis that can be performed readily with the dynamic evaluation software included on many CT systems is described below. However, the use of curve-fitting procedures, which unfortunately may not be available on standard software packages, will produce more accurate results (see the discussion on advanced processing below).

The method uses the maximal gradient method. Time–attenuation data from a ROI over a major vessel gives the peak arterial enhancement and the maximal gradient can be determined by linear interpolation of the tissue time–attenuation points. Table 5.2 gives example time–attenuation data from a liver study with ROIs over aorta, spleen and liver. The maximal rate of enhancement of the spleen occurs between 13 and 16 s. The enhancement over this time is 21 HU giving a rate of 21/3 or 7 HU/s. Dividing by the peak arterial attenuation of 250 HU gives a splenic perfusion of 0.028 ml/s/ml. Multiplying by 60 converts this to 1.68 ml/min/ml.

Table 5.2
Example of time–attenuation data from a liver study

Time (s)	Change in attenuation (HU)		
	Aorta	Spleen	Liver
0	0	0	0
7	4	0	1
10	30	0	0
13	181	0	0
16	250	21	2
19	168	37	2
24	40	48	5
29	28	45	7
34	37	32	17
41.5	43	29	20

To determine hepatic perfusion, the time of peak splenic enhancement can be used to separate arterial and portal phases of hepatic enhancement. In the example in Table 5.2, this occurs at 24 s. The maximal rate of liver enhancement before this time occurs between 16 and 19 s giving a slope of 2 HU over 3 s (0.67 HU/s). Dividing by peak arterial enhancement (250 HU) and converting to minutes gives hepatic arterial perfusion of 0.16 ml/min/ml. Similarly, the maximal rate of liver enhancement occurs between 29 and 34 s giving a slope of 10 HU over 5 s (2 HU/s) corresponding to a portal perfusion of 0.48 ml/min/ml (indirect method; see Chapter 6).

ADVANCED PROCESSING AND PERFUSION IMAGES

Many of the more advanced methods of analysis may not be available on the dynamic evaluation software. For ROI analysis, this can be overcome by transferring the data to a commercially available spreadsheet program customized to perform the appropriate analysis. Generation of parametric images, including perfusion images, will require dedicated software such as that developed at Addenbrooke's Hospital, Cambridge, UK.

Curve-fitting procedures are of great importance in obtaining accurate results either from ROI analysis or perfusion imaging. A gamma variate or cubic spline fit to the arterial time–attenuation curve will improve the accuracy in determining peak vascular enhancement. A gamma-variate function is also required to determine the area under the arterial curve corrected for recirculation as required for the Mullani–Gould analysis. Applying a curve-fitting procedure to the tissue time–attenuation data may also produce more reliable perfusion measurements. A cubic spline fit using three or more points of the upslope can be used to determine the maximal rate of enhancement when using the gradient method whereas peak tissue enhancement, as required for Mullani–Gould analysis, can be determined from a gamma-variate fit. Reproducibility tests will confirm that line fits are repeatable and that the values obtained are not spurious. In some circumstances, curve-fitting tissue time–attenuation data can exaggerate the effects of noise, particularly when measuring low-perfusion values from very small ROIs or individual pixels.

The method for determining hepatic portal perfusion from the maximal gradient of the late-enhancement phase, as described above, provides an indirect measure only. A more rigorous approach is to normalize the liver enhancement with respect to the portal vein. If a portal (or, if this is not possible, splenic) vein time–attenuation curve can be constructed, a gamma-variate fit can be performed and the peak enhancement divided into the late-phase gradient of the liver curve. This technique can be further improved by firstly removing any arterial component from the liver time–attenuation data. This can be achieved by using a time–attenuation curve derived from a ROI over the spleen as a template for hepatic arterial perfusion. First, hepatic arterial and splenic perfusion are calculated using the gradient technique and the ratio of the two perfusion values is determined. The baseline-subtracted splenic time–attenuation curve is then multiplied by this ratio. This produces a scaled-down splenic curve which is then subtracted from the initial 'raw' liver curve, thereby removing the arterial component. The peak gradient of the resultant curve is then divided by peak portal or splenic venous enhancement to measure hepatic portal perfusion. This analysis method, despite its complexity, produces reproducible and physiologically appropriate values.

Identification of the vascular ROI can be made easier by reference to a functional image displaying maximal enhancement values. This is particularly useful with brain studies where no large vessels are available. Use of an edge detection algorithm can further improve the quality of data from the vascular ROI by minimizing partial volume effects. An algorithm we have found effective identifies the most enhancing pixel within a ROI and then defines as 'vascular' all pixels with peak enhancement within 10% and time of peak enhancement within 3 s of that of the most enhancing pixel. Within the brain, the most enhancing pixels may be within a venous rather than an arterial structure due to small arteries suffering partial volume effects. In our experience, in these circumstances it is better to use a venous rather than an arterial ROI. Although this will underestimate peak vascular enhancement, the error will be smaller than using an arterial ROI and therefore will produce the most accurate result.

Once the arterial ROI is determined, perfusion images can be generated automatically by computer analysis of time–attenuation data from corresponding pixels from each of the series of images. For images of hepatic arterial and portal perfusion, data from a splenic ROI are required from which the time of peak splenic enhancement is determined. This time point is used to separate arterial and portal phases. Arterial perfusion must be calculated from the maximum slope before this time point as, in the normal liver, the maximal rate of enhancement occurs in the portal phase. Portal perfusion images can be generated using the time–attenuation data from individual liver pixels after the time of peak splenic enhancement.

Most modern CT systems produce images using a 512×512 or 1024×1024 matrix. Compression of the original image data to a 256×256 matrix reduces photon noise and allows rapid calculation without significantly degrading spatial resolution. In some cases, the perfusion images can be improved by additional spatial smoothing. The requirement for smoothing depends on the signal-to-noise ratio. On account of the relatively low-perfusion values and effects of attenuation from the skull, brain studies particularly benefit from spatial smoothing (see Chapter 2).

If perfusion within the organ under study is exceptionally low, perfusion values from individual pixels can be spuriously high as the computer algorithm may be more likely to detect noise or even slight motion artefacts. In these circumstances, it can be useful to predetermine the time of maximal enhancement rate by reference to a more highly perfused organ in which these effects will be negligible. If, for instance, the maximal rate of enhancement for the reference organ occurs between 16 and 19 s, then the slope of the time–density curve from the poorly perfused tissue over the same period is used to calculate perfusion. This 'forcing' technique may be particularly useful for livers with very low or absent arterial perfusion. Often, liver time–density curves demonstrate a small 'blip' very early on due to back-flow of contrast medium from the right atrium via hepatic veins to the liver parenchyma (see liver time–attenuation data in Table 5.2). If this effect produces a rate of enhancement greater than that of the true hepatic arterial phase, automated analysis may falsely identify the first increase for use in calculating perfusion. The forced method of analysis prevents this error.

Separate measurement of perfusion within the lymphatic cords and matrix of the spleen can be useful in the evaluation of portal hypertension (see Chapter 7). Rather than attempting to define very small ROIs based on the inhomogeneous enhancement pattern of the spleen, the two components of splenic perfusion can be determined statistically. The pixels within a larger splenic ROI are divided into two populations on the basis of their time to maximal enhancement. The threshold that separates the early enhancing pixels that correspond to lymphatic cords from the late enhancing pixels of the splenic matrix is determined iteratively such that the standard errors of the two populations is minimal. This method also benefits from consistency as there is no opportunity for operator error.

REGION OF INTEREST ANALYSIS OR PERFUSION IMAGES?

Region of interest analysis is most appropriate for tissues that are generally homogeneous and also benefits from a much lower sensitivity to noise. Thus, with ROI analysis alone, it may be possible to use smaller amounts of contrast medium with the benefit of improved bolus geometry as discussed above. On the other hand, construction of a ROI using conventional CT images requires assumptions about areas of high or low perfusion to be made from anatomical features. For instance, within the kidney there are no clearly defined criteria that separate cortex and medulla. Thus, when there are regional variations of perfusion within an organ, bias may be introduced when there is a discrepancy between anatomical boundaries and zones of differing perfusion. The construction of perfusion images avoids this problem as there is no prejudgement required as to areas of high or low perfusion. The disadvantage of perfusion images is the increased noise introduced when using pixel by pixel analysis. A compromise can be achieved by first producing a perfusion image which is used to define ROIs from which the final perfusion values are obtained. The effects of noise inherent within the functional image are avoided and, although not entirely free of bias, zones of differing perfusion are defined more appropriately by using functional rather than anatomical criteria.

Chapter 6

PERFUSION CT: NORMAL ORGANS

K. Miles and M. Blomley

KIDNEY

Anatomy and physiology

The kidney is one of the most highly perfused organs. Together, the two kidneys receive approximately 25% of the cardiac output whilst comprising less than 0.5% of total body weight. Although typically each kidney is supplied by a single artery and vein, multiple arteries or veins are common normal variants.

Within the kidney itself, there is a close relationship between vascular anatomy and the structure of the nephron resulting in intrarenal variations in perfusion. Differences in circulation between renal cortex and medulla were first demonstrated in 1947 by Trueta *et al.* [1] using angiography. This was subsequently amplified by angiographic studies [2] revealing further differences between outer and inner medulla in dogs.

The intrarenal circulation is summarized in Figure 6.1. The interlobar arteries form arcuate arteries at the corticomedullary junction. The cortex is supplied by

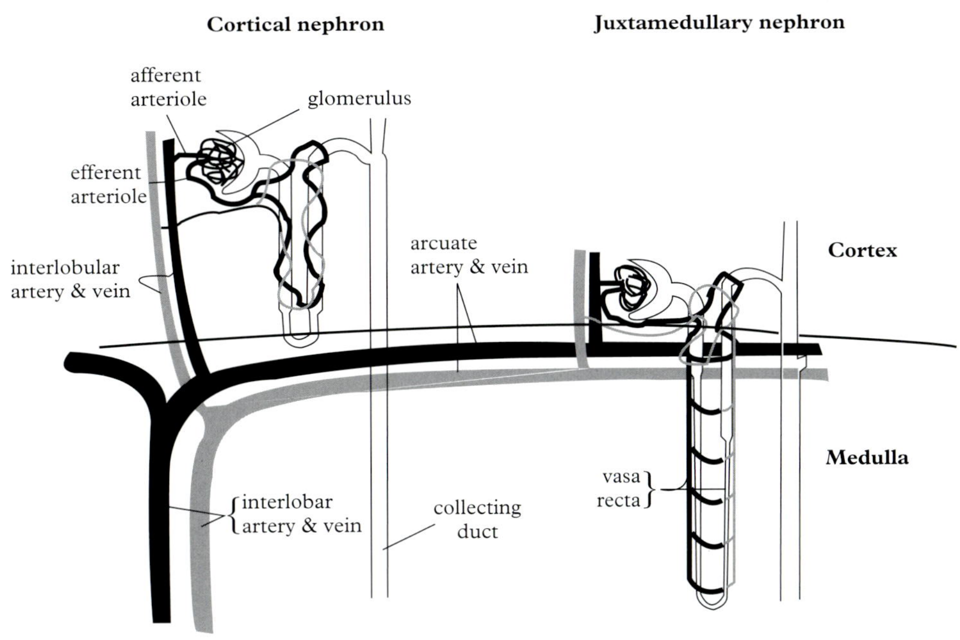

Figure 6.1 Renal circulation.

the interlobular arteries which arise from the arcuate arteries. The medulla is supplied by the vasa recta which are formed from branches of the efferent arterioles of the juxtamedullary nephrons alone. The medulla is therefore perfused entirely by blood from the inner cortex.

Intrarenal variations in perfusion can be demonstrated by compartmental analysis of wash-out curves following intra-arterial injection of inert radioactive gases such as xenon-133 and krypton-85. A series of exponential curves is derived, each said to correspond to a particular territory. Unfortunately, different studies have reported variable numbers of compartments and the exact anatomical region related to a specific compartment has not been reliably established. However, autoradiography and gamma-camera techniques have suggested that the first exponential corresponds to the renal cortex. The use of such techniques in man yields a cortical perfusion within the range of 4–5 ml/min/ml and medullary perfusion 0.7–1.5 ml/min/ml [3].

An alternative approach to studying intrarenal variations in perfusion has been the use of deconvolutional analysis of data from conventional radioisotope renography using iodohippuran and a gamma-camera [4]. Deconvolution yields a spectrum of transit times for passage of tracer through the kidney. By considering data from an outer renal region, the spectrum of transit times relating to cortical nephrons is determined. Subtraction of this spectrum from one derived from a combined corticomedullary region gives the medullary spectrum. As uptake of iodohippuran is dependent upon renal perfusion, the relative sizes of cortical and medullary spectra determine the corticomedullary perfusion ratio. A ratio of approximately 4:1 is obtained in normal subjects. Absolute perfusion values cannot be derived using this technique.

CT measurements of renal perfusion

Early reports of computed tomography (CT) evaluation of renal perfusion used semiquantitative measures only. In 1981, Ishikawa *et al.* [5] described the time–attenuation curves of normal kidneys and the time taken for aortic and renal cortical time–attenuation curves to cross, typically 45 s, was proposed as an indicator of renal perfusion. Probst *et al.* [6] used a comparison of peak renal enhancement between the two kidneys as a measure of relative renal perfusion. In normal subjects, this peak occurred 7–8 s after that of the aorta with a difference between normal kidneys of 2.7 ± 2.2 HU. The ratio of the slopes of time–attenuation curves from renal cortex or medulla and aorta were used by Jansen *et al.* [7] to generate a perfusion index akin to that frequently used in nuclear medicine techniques.

The first report of absolute quantification of renal perfusion using CT was by Jaschke *et al.* in 1987 [8]. Using an ultra-fast electron beam CT system with 50 ms exposures and a repetition rate of up to 17 per second, they measured renal cortical perfusion in dogs at 5.7 ml/min/ml. In a later report, the same group reported inner medullary perfusion in the dog to be 0.45 ml/min/ml [9]. In both studies, a first-pass method was used with analysis based on the Fick principle. The technique required time–attenuation measurements, not only from aorta and kidney, but also from the renal vein, limiting the technique to studies at the level of the renal hilum. The venous data were used to determine the quantity of contrast material leaving the kidney within the time interval of the measurement and it was assumed that flow through the medulla did not contribute to the venous outflow during this period. Cortical perfusion measurements correlated well with values determined using radioactive microspheres.

Early attempts to measure regional renal perfusion in man using conventional CT equipment [10] gave normal values for cortex and medulla of 2.5 ml/min/ml and 1.1 ml/min/ml, respectively, using the gradient method of analysis (Chapter 4). However, the poor temporal sampling afforded by the CT equipment used (i.e. a 6 s data acquisition every 8 s) caused underestimation of the slope of the cortical time–attenuation curve and therefore values for cortical perfusion that were too low.

The use of faster imaging sequences that are possible with modern slip-ring CT systems (e.g. 1 s exposures repeated every 3–5 s) overcomes this problem and yields cortical perfusion values in man of 4.7 ml/min/ml with medullary perfusion of 1.1 ml/min/ml [11]; values close to those previously obtained with radioactive xenon. Similar results were later obtained in man using ultrafast (electron beam) CT and rapid (less than 2.5 s) boluses of contrast medium [12].

In addition to region of interest (ROI) analysis, parametric images of renal perfusion can be produced (Figure 6.2). These have an advantage over ROI analysis in which regions are created with reference to anatomical features, thus requiring assumptions as to regions of high and low perfusion to be made prior to analysis. The high spatial resolution of the images also enables direct anatomical localization of regions of high and low perfusion, confirming the cortex as the most highly perfused zone.

In most cases, the transition between the high cortical perfusion and lower medullary perfusion is gradual, either due to spatial overlap of physiologically

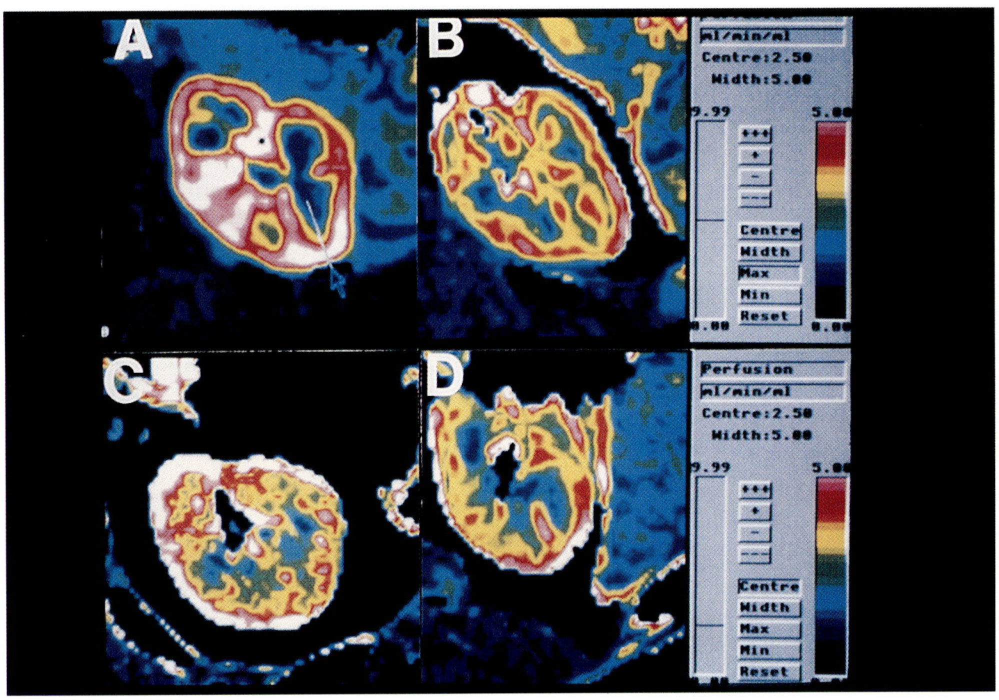

Figure 6.2 CT perfusion images from four human kidneys (pink: 5 ml/min/ml).

distinct compartments or partial volume effects. Likewise, functional images demonstrate no difference in perfusion between outer and inner medulla, suggesting that the separate medullary compartments inferred from inert gas wash-out are not anatomically distinct.

The information derived from perfusion CT of the kidney is of great value as it allows direct visualization of intrarenal variations in perfusion with such high spatial resolution and absolute quantification of perfusion values.

PANCREAS

Anatomy and physiology

The pancreas is supplied with blood from three main sources:

(1) the superior pancreaticoduodenal artery, an end artery of the gastroduodenal artery, supplies the head of the gland and part of the body and uncinate process;
(2) the body and tail are supplied by branches of the splenic artery;
(3) the inferior pancreaticoduoenal artery arises from the superior mesenteric artery to supply part of the uncinate process. Venous drainage is largely into the splenic vein.

Despite its importance to the endocrine and exocrine functions of the pancreas, measurement of pancreatic perfusion in man has proved extremely difficult. Canine perfusion has been measured using thermocouples, isotope fractionation (e.g. microspheres), hydrogen desaturation and the wash-out of radioactive inert gases. All of these methods are invasive and have yielded varying results between techniques and between anaesthetized and ambulant dogs [13]. Taking all methods into account, canine pancreatic perfusion lies between 0.1 and 2.0 ml/min/ml.

Attempts have been made to measure pancreatic perfusion in man using radiolabelled water and positron emission tomography (PET) [14]. However, the spatial resolution of PET cannot allow the pancreas and the many surrounding vascular structures to be separated with any certainty.

CT measurements of pancreatic perfusion

CT perfusion imaging has enabled non-invasive measurement of pancreatic perfusion in man which has hitherto proven impossible. The high spatial resolution of the technique allows clear distinction between pancreas and surrounding vessels and evaluation of regional changes in perfusion. Using the gradient method of calculating perfusion (see Chapter 4), perfusion CT gives a mean pancreatic perfusion in the normal human pancreas of 1.5 ml/min/ml (range 1.25–1.66 ml/min/ml) [15]. CT perfusion images demonstrate even perfusion throughout the head, body and tail (Figure 6.3).

SPLEEN

Anatomy and physiology

The spleen is essentially a lymphatic organ but it is the only organ of the lymphatic system to filter the blood. It selectively weakens abnormal or senescent

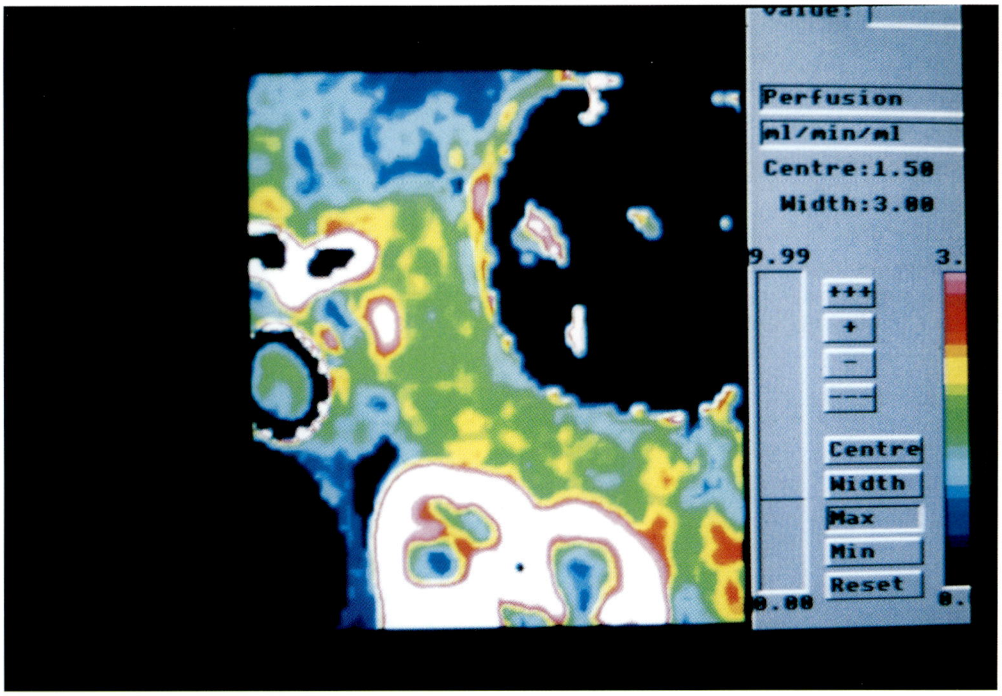

Figure 6.3
CT perfusion image of a normal human pancreas (pink: 3 ml/min/ml).

red cells prior to their destruction in the circulation — a process known as 'conditioning'. The spleen receives its blood supply via the splenic artery, a branch of the coeliac trunk. The splenic vein drains into the portal venous system and thus changes in portal venous pressure secondary to liver disease are transmitted to the spleen resulting in changes in splenic perfusion. Structurally, the spleen comprises white pulp and red pulp. The white pulp is a sheath of lymphatic tissue surrounding the arteries and is thickened in places to form lymphatic nodules. The red pulp occupies most of the parenchyma and is the site of the organ's filtration function.

The microcirculation of the spleen and its relationship to the organ's internal structure and filtration function have been of much interest and is diagrammatically summarized in Figure 6.4. Studies of the wash-out of radiolabelled plasma from the spleen demonstrate a biexponential curve implying two vascular pathways — one slow and one fast. Similar studies using radiolabelled red cells demonstrate a third compartment, not seen with plasma studies. This represents sequestration of red cells within the spleen. It is estimated that about 90% of the splenic blood flow is via the fast pathway with 10% passing through the slow pathway [16].

The morphological counterparts for these physiological compartments have been sought using corrosion casting and *in vivo* microscopy. Such studies indicate that blood flows through the white pulp and then the red pulp in series. Within the lymphoid follicles, capillaries may connect directly with the venous sinuses. This is known as the 'closed system'. Alternatively, some capillaries terminate in the marginal zone of the lymphoid follicle close to open-ended venous sinuses whilst others open into the reticular meshwork of the red pulp. Blood then passes from the reticular meshwork into the venous sinuses through

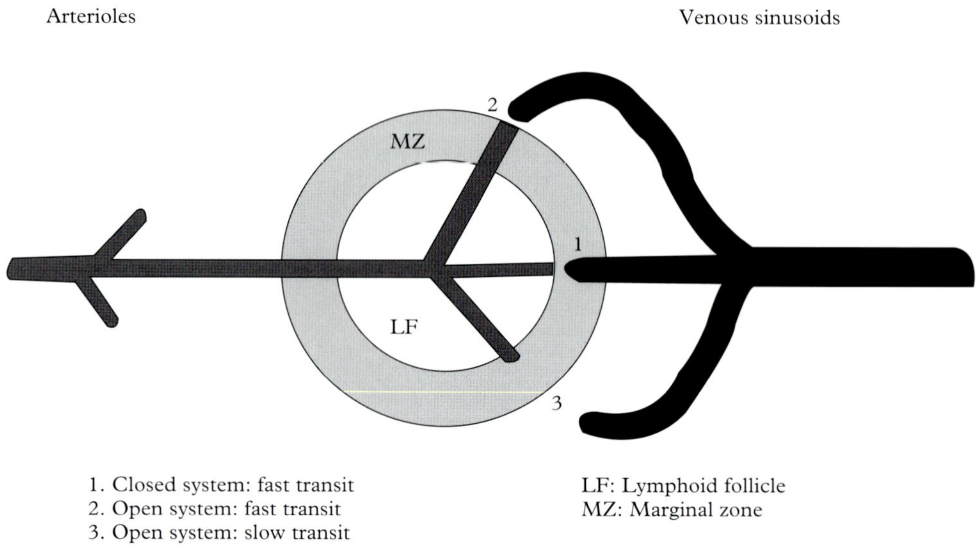

Figure 6.4
Diagrammatic representation of the splenic microcirculation.

endothelial slits. These latter two routes are known as the 'open system'. The fast-flow pathway comprises the direct capillary–venous connections (closed system) and the route via the open-ended capillaries in the marginal zone (part of the open system). The slow-flow pathway is via the reticular meshwork of the red pulp (part of the open system) and it is this pathway that is associated with the filtration function of the spleen.

Global splenic perfusion can be determined from the wash-out of radioactive inert gases (xenon-133 and krypton-85) using either intra-arterial injection or inhalation. Such techniques give values of between 0.96 and 1.19 ml/min/g for the normal human spleen [17–21] (Figure 6.5). Methods using radiolabelled blood cells such as platelets or erythrocytes give different results due to sequestration of the cells within the spleen and cannot be considered equivalent to techniques using plasma markers, including perfusion CT.

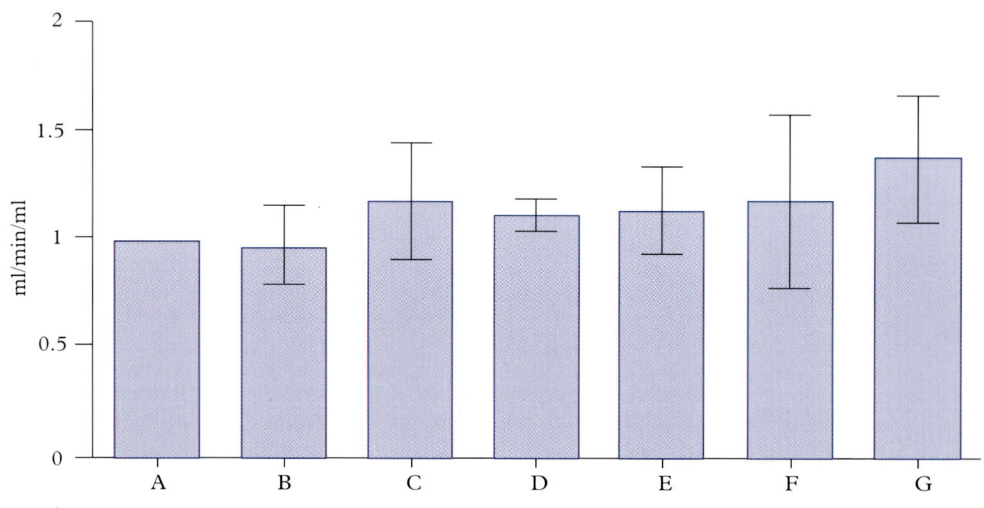

Figure 6.5
Normal splenic perfusion values as determined using inert-gas techniques and functional CT. A, Williams *et al.* [17]; B, Gitlin *et al.* [18]; C, Ueda *et al.* [19]; D, Huchzermeyer *et al.* [20]; E, Takahashi *et al.* [21]; F, IGE 8800; G, Siemens.

CT perfusion studies of the spleen

CT measurements of global perfusion in the normal human spleen [11,22,23] have all produced similar results despite using different calculation algorithms and different CT systems, including one study using ultra-fast CT [24]. CT values for normal splenic perfusion range between 1.2 and 1.4 ml/min/ml and are in close agreement with those obtained using inert gas wash-out techniques (Figure 6.5) although CT measurements tend to be slightly higher. One reason for this discrepancy is that CT expresses perfusion in units of ml/min/ml whereas inert gas techniques use ml/min/g. The density of the spleen is approximately 1.05 g/ml and therefore CT can be expected to overestimate perfusion by 5% as compared with inert-gas techniques. Furthermore, due to the high affinity of inert gases for lipids, such techniques are affected by the fat content of tissues, whereas perfusion CT is unaffected. In the case of the spleen, this error could be in the region of 10% [20].

The use of CT to generate parametric images of splenic perfusion enables direct visualization of regional variations in perfusion within the spleen (Figure 6.6a). Hitherto this injection has not been possible using other techniques due to inadequate spatial resolution. Heterogeneous enhancement of the spleen following intravenous contrast medium injection has long been recognized as a normal finding both with CT and magnetic resonance imaging (MRI). Glazer *et al.* [24] proposed that this may be due to regional variations in perfusion, a fact confirmed by CT perfusion images. Generation of an additional parametric image displaying time to peak enhancement provides further interesting information about intrasplenic haemodynamics (Figure 6.6b). A pattern comprising regions of early and late enhancement is seen. By comparing perfusion and time to peak images it can be seen that the regions of high perfusion correspond to the regions of early enhancement and vice versa.

The pixels within the spleen can be divided into two populations based on their time to peak enhancement. A statistical method that avoids operator bias divides the two populations iteratively such that the sum of the variances of the two populations is the minimum [23]. Within a series of normal spleens, 77% of the pixels fell within the early enhancing population with a mean time to peak enhancement of 24.5 s. On average, the remaining 33% of pixels reached peak enhancement 9.3 s later.

Time to peak enhancement can be considered an indicator of transit time and therefore the above process divides the spleen into fast and slow transit regions, broadly equivalent to the two pathways found on plasma wash-out studies and their respective morphological counterparts. Thus, CT perfusion imaging can separately measure perfusion within the lymphoid follicles (early enhancing regions) and the splenic matrix (late enhancing regions). For the normal human spleen, these values have been found to be 1.44 ml/min/ml and 1.24 ml/min/ml respectively [23].

LIVER

Anatomy and physiology

The circulation of the liver is complicated by its dual blood supply. Arterial blood reaches the liver via the hepatic artery, a branch of the coeliac trunk. The portal

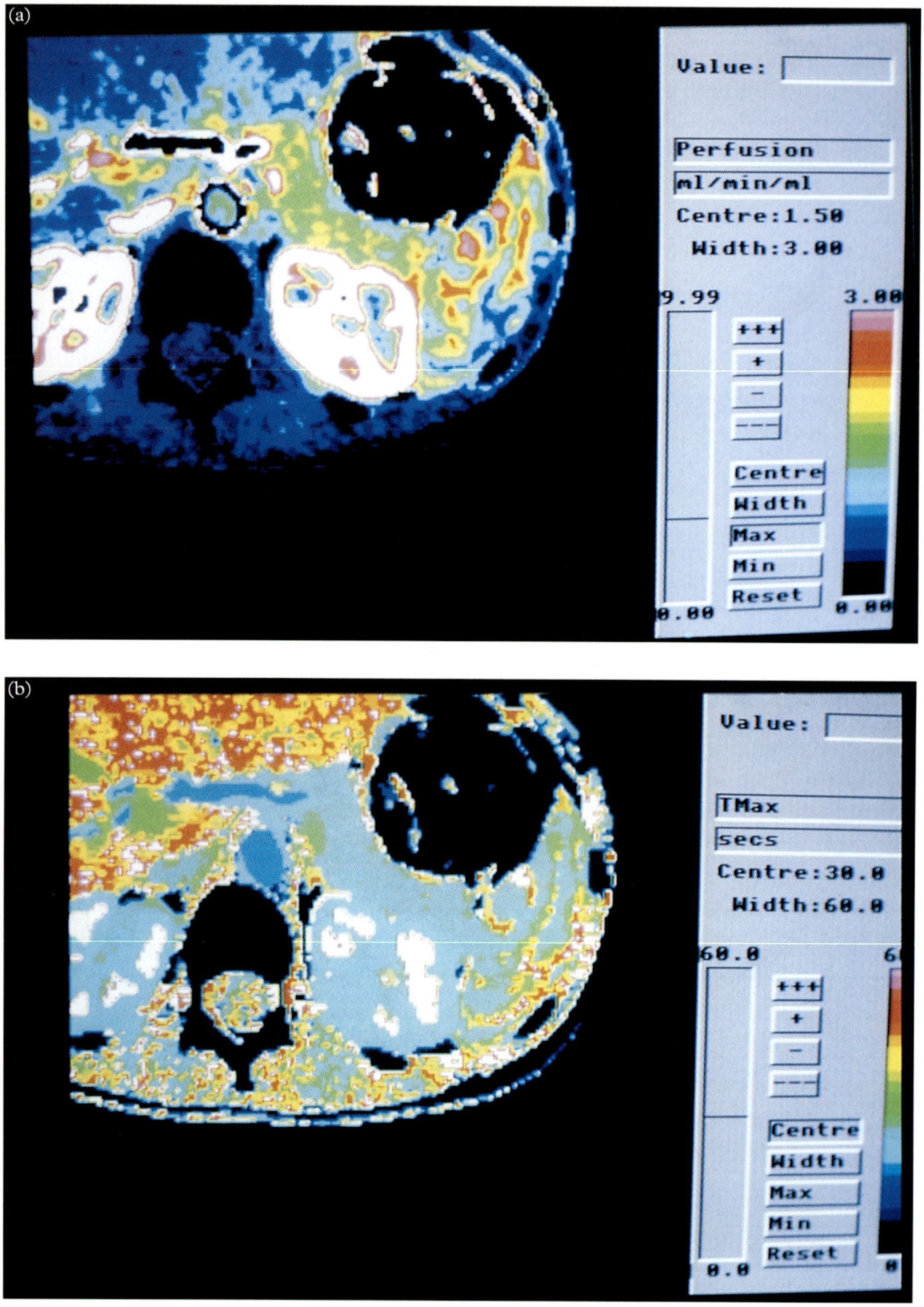

Figure 6.6
Perfusion image (a) and time to peak enhancement image (b) of a normal spleen (blue: low perfusion/early enhancement; pink: high perfusion (3 ml/min/ml)/late enhancement).

venous supply comprises blood returning from the spleen and gut via the superior mesenteric and splenic veins which join to form the portal vein. Venous drainage is via the three hepatic veins into the inferior vena cava shortly before its entry into the right atrium.

Arterial and portal blood mix within the sinusoids of the liver. This arrangement provides a mechanism for the reciprocal relationship that has been observed between arterial and portal blood flow. A drop in portal perfusion is associated with increased arterial perfusion and vice versa. The mechanism is independent of neuronal control, occurring in the transplanted liver, for example, and appears to be a simple impedance effect [25,26].

There is evidence of macroscopic regional variations in perfusion within the liver [27,28] but with no consistent pattern. Some reports also describe a preferential intrahepatic distribution of blood from the spleen [28,29] but this has been the source of much controversy.

Although global liver blood flow can be assessed by the blood clearance of hepatically extracted tracers, such as bromosulphthalein and indocyanine, determination of hepatic perfusion (flow per unit mass or volume) in man has relied on inert-gas wash-out techniques. The gas can be administered by one of a number of routes but usually splenic injection is used. The technique measures combined arterial and portal perfusion and the mean normal value in man is 1.11 ml/min/g [30]. Until the development of perfusion CT techniques, direct measurement of the separate arterial and portal components of hepatic perfusion has not been possible. However, the ratio of arterial to portal perfusion can be determined using a number of nuclear medicine techniques including dynamic colloid scintigraphy. These indicate that the arterial supply contributes about 25% of total hepatic perfusion. Thus, extrapolating from both techniques, absolute arterial perfusion is approximately 0.3 ml/min/ml.

CT measurements of hepatic perfusion

The dual blood supply to the liver results in a biphasic pattern of hepatic enhancement following intravenous contrast medium injection (Figure 6.7). In the normal liver, the early arterial enhancement is less than the later portal enhancement, reflecting the greater portal perfusion. This biphasic pattern also prevents use of the Mullani–Gould method for calculating perfusion as it is impossible to determine the peak enhancement due to each phase separately. One approach has been to apply the gradient method to each phase separately,

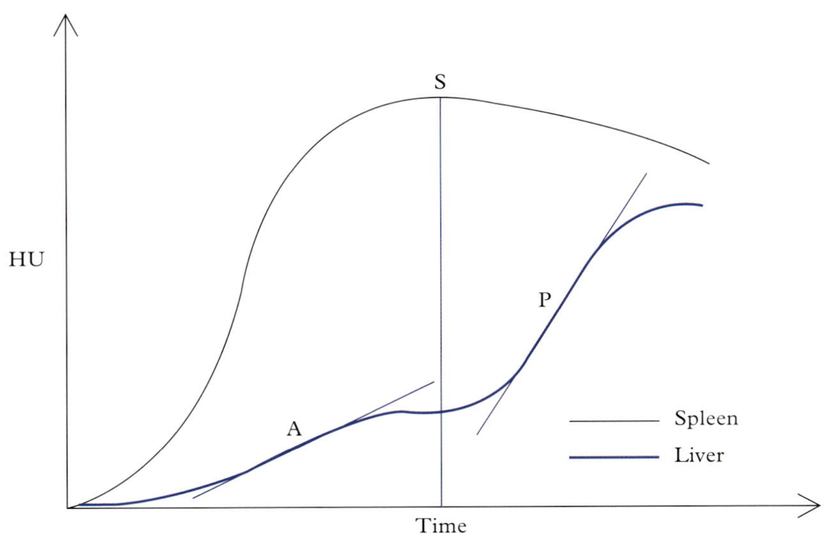

Figure 6.7 Stylized spleen and liver time–attenuation curves. (A) time of maximal slope in arterial phase. (P) time of maximal slope in portal phase. (S) time of peak splenic enhancement.

Table 6.1
Times of maximal arterial and portal slopes of liver time–attenuation curves and their relationship to the time of peak splenic enhancement

Time	Mean (s)	Range (s)
Time of maximal slope in arterial phase (A)	15.3	10.5–25.9
Time of maximal slope in portal phase (P)	30.6	20.7–36.8
Time of peak splenic enhancement (S)	24.4	15.4–33.4
Time between maximum arterial slope and splenic peak (A-S)	9.1	1.8–22.9
Time between splenic peak and maximum portal slope (S-P)	6.2	1.0–21.3
Time between maximum arterial and portal slopes (A-P)	15.3	4.0–26.2

using the time to peak splenic enhancement to distinguish the two phases. Table 6.1 gives the temporal characteristics from a group of liver time–attenuation curves following a rapid bolus of 50 ml of contrast medium [31]. The arterial and portal slopes are well separated and therefore errors in determining the time of peak splenic enhancement are unlikely to affect liver-perfusion measurements. This method provides only an *indirect measure* of portal perfusion and significantly underestimates true portal perfusion due to spreading of the bolus and loss of contrast medium into the extracellular space during passage through the spleen. An alternative approach provides a more *direct measure* by using time–attenuation data from a ROI over portal or splenic vein, rather than aorta, as the input function for the portal component of the liver enhancement [31]. However, the portion of liver that can be studied by this method is limited to those slices that contain portal or splenic vein. Functional images of arterial and portal perfusion are more readily obtained using the indirect method for portal assessment. Example images from a normal liver are given in Figure 6.8.

Computed tomography measurements of arterial perfusion in the normal liver give mean values of approximately 0.17 ml/min/ml [31,33]. Using the indirect method, the mean value of portal perfusion in the normal liver is 0.41 ml/min/ml and combined arterial and portal (total) perfusion is 0.58 ml/min/ml [31]. The ratios of arterial to total perfusion, equivalent to the hepatic perfusion index (HPI) used in nuclear medicine, determined using this technique have been validated against dynamic colloid scintigraphy [31] with CT values in the normal liver of 0.32. The direct method produces more physiological values of 0.93 ml/min/ml for portal perfusion and 1.12 for total perfusion [33].

Macroscopic regional variations in hepatic perfusion can also be seen with CT perfusion imaging (Table 6.2). Left-lobe perfusion is more variable than that of

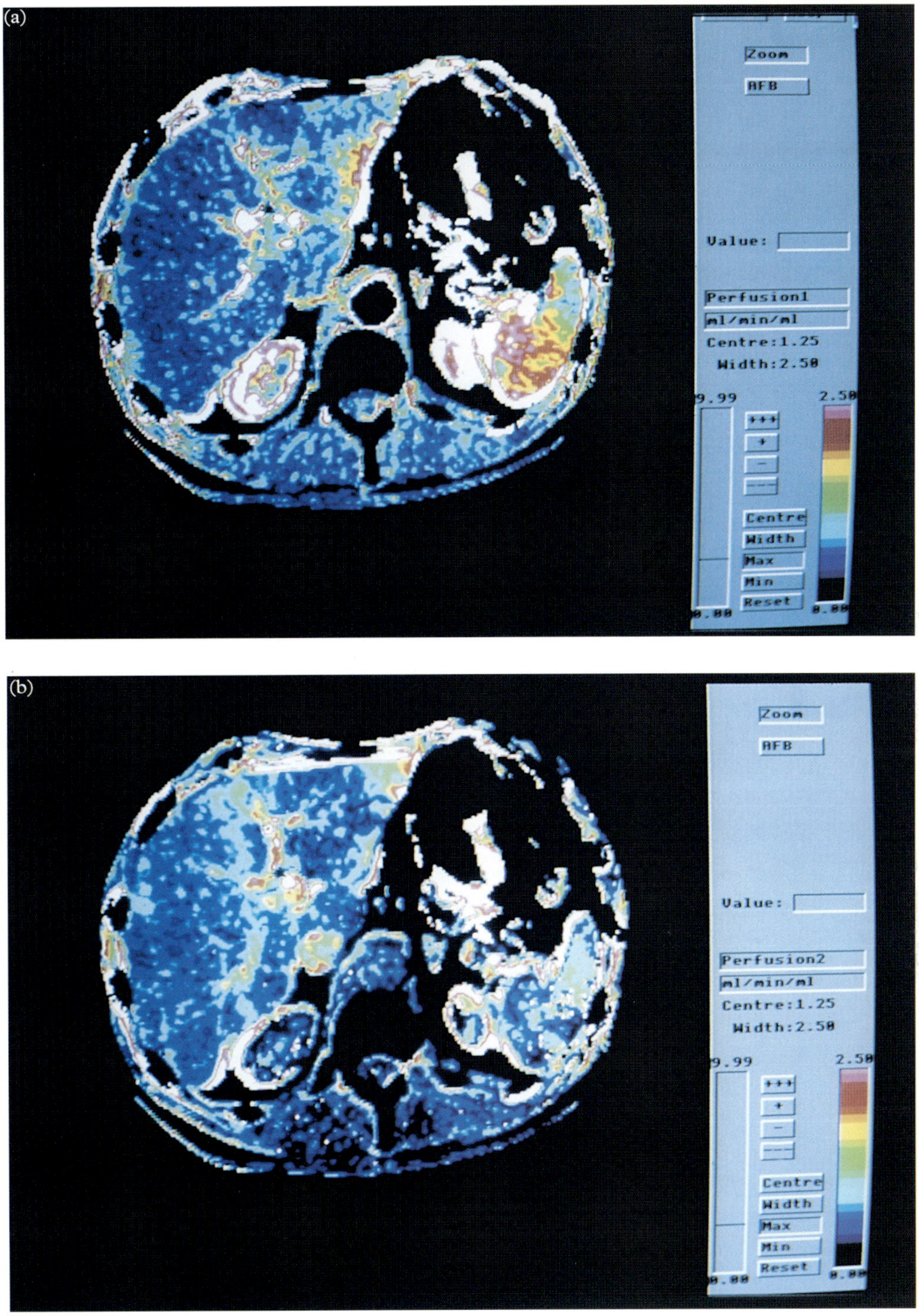

Figure 6.8
Functional images of (a) arterial and (b) indirect portal perfusion in a normal liver (pink: 2.5 ml/min/ml).

the right lobe. In general, arterial perfusion is found to be higher in the left lobe but this is associated with lower portal perfusion reflecting the reciprocal relationship between the two circulations. Thus, differences in combined arterial and portal perfusion between the lobes are less marked, although there is a slight trend for higher combined values in the left lobe. The greater left-lobe arterial

Parameter	Right lobe	Left lobe
Arterial perfusion (ml/min/ml)	0.17	0.37
Indirect portal perfusion (ml/min/ml)	0.41	0.33
Combined arterial and indirect portal perfusion (ml/min/ml)	0.58	0.70
Hepatic perfusion index (HPI)	0.29	0.53

Table 6.2
Hepatic perfusion values for right and left lobes (gradient method of calculation)

perfusion is also reflected in increased values of HPI. When large, differences in perfusion between the lobes can be appreciated on the conventional CT images as transient differences in lobar attenuation (Figure 6.9). In addition, in a group comprising patients with normal and abnormal livers, a correlation has been observed between right-lobe portal perfusion and splenic perfusion but no correlation is seen on the left [32].

BRAIN

Anatomy and physiology

Blood is carried to the brain via two internal carotid and two vertebral arteries with a small contribution from the anterior spinal artery to the medulla. The

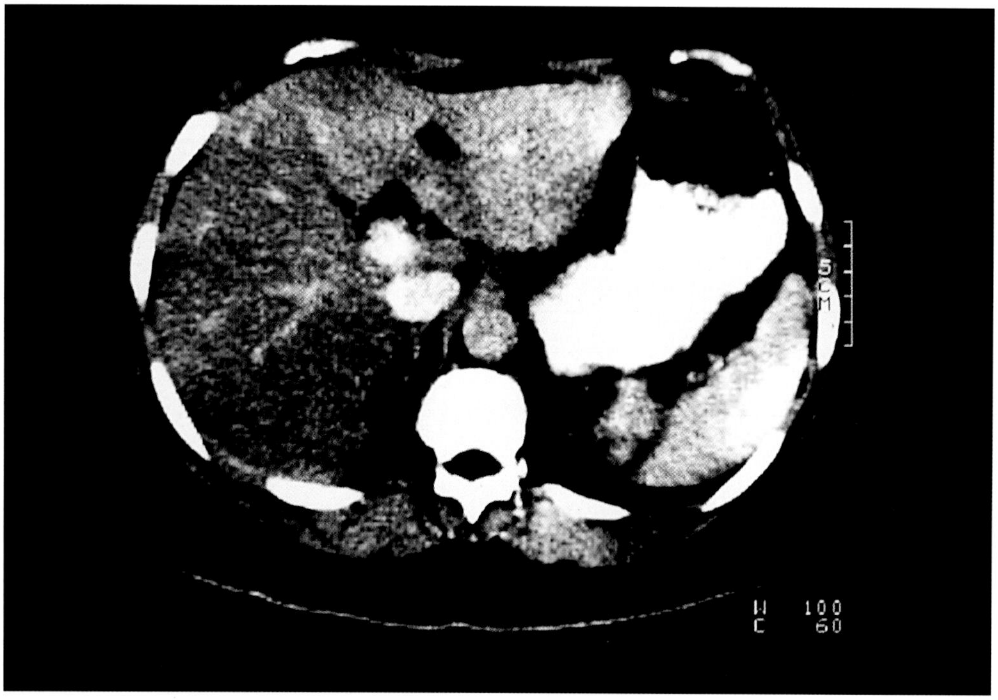

Figure 6.9
Image from a single-location dynamic sequence to study liver perfusion. Greater arterial perfusion in the left lobe is seen as a transient difference in lobar attenuation.

vertebral arteries unite to form the basilar artery from which the cerebellum is supplied by inferior and superior cerebellar arteries. The basilar artery also supplies the brainstem and divides to form the posterior cerebral arteries which supply the occipital lobes and inferior portions of the temporal lobes. They also contribute posterior communicating arteries to the circle of Willis which is completed by the anterior and middle cerebral arteries, formed by division of the internal carotid artery and the anterior communicating artery. The anterior cerebral artery supplies the superior aspect of the parietal lobe, the anterior and inferior aspects of the frontal lobe, and the medial aspects of both. The middle cerebral artery supplies the lateral aspects of these two lobes and the remainder of the temporal lobe. Under normal conditions, there is very little crossover between the two sides via the circle of Willis.

Although activation of specific brain regions produces a local increase in blood flow, total brain blood flow is generally constant. Factors affecting global cerebral perfusion include the arterial and venous pressures at brain level, intracranial pressure and the degree of vasoconstriction or dilatation of cerebral arterioles. The arterioles are particularly sensitive to carbon dioxide which causes vasodilation — an effect that can be used diagnostically to reveal critical stenoses within arteries supplying the brain.

Quantitative measurements of cerebral perfusion have been made by various techniques that use diffusible tracers. These include scintillation probe or emission tomographic studies with radioactive xenon, xenon CT and ^{15}O water with PET. Single-photon emission computed tomography (SPECT) yields relative perfusion only. Functional MRI techniques, such as deoxyhaemoglobin imaging, generally measure changes in cerebral perfusion rather than providing absolute quantification.

Interestingly, cerebral perfusion values are lower than those for many abdominal organs. Although some variation in perfusion values is seen amongst the results with diffusible techniques, generally normal grey matter (cortical) perfusion is found to be between 0.7 and 0.9 ml/min/g. However, ^{15}O water with PET yields lower values at 0.55 ml/min/g. Values for white matter fall between 0.2 and 0.3 ml/min/g but tomographic radioactive xenon techniques give values of 0.59 ml/min/g [34] as a uniform partition coefficient for all brain tissue is assumed. Some variation in perfusion between different brain regions has been reported but these tend to be technique dependent. This may result from differences in the environment under which the techniques are performed leading to variations in the amount of brain activation in different brain regions.

CT measurements of cerebral perfusion

Dynamic CT techniques for assessing perfusion with iodinated contrast media use a first-pass technique during which the contrast medium behaves as a non-diffusible tracer. Axel proposed a dynamic CT method for measuring cerebral perfusion in 1980 [35] based on determination of transit times from time–attenuation curves. However, due to technical difficulties in obtaining an adequate arterial time–attenuation curve within the cranium, he suggested that the reciprocal of transit time could be more readily used as a measure of relative

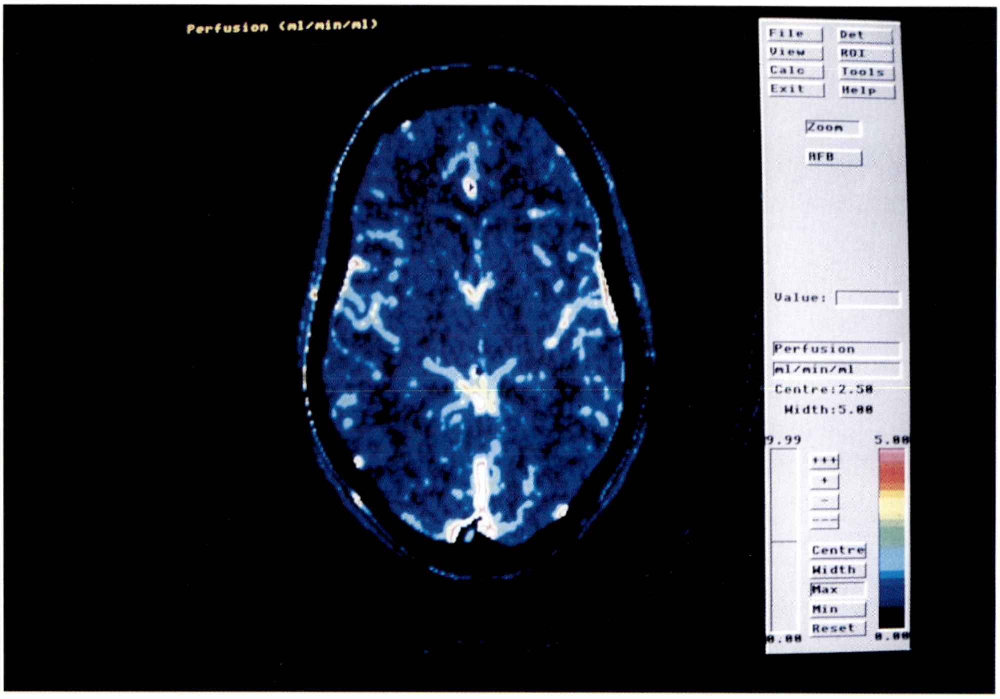

Figure 6.10
CT cerebral perfusion image of normal brain (gradient method; pink: 5 ml/min/ml).

cerebral perfusion. The following year, Axel and co-workers published a functional image of relative cerebral perfusion by performing his analysis pixel by pixel [36]. In 1983, Axel proposed an alternative method for measuring cerebral perfusion by determination of absolute transit time through constrained deconvolution [37]. By assuming a fractional blood volume for brain tissue of 5%, this method produced a value 1.15 ml/min/ml for cerebral grey matter, somewhat higher than accepted values obtained with diffusible tracers.

Peak cerebral enhancement following bolus administration of contrast can also be used as a measure of relative cerebral perfusion, based on the Mullani–Gould method of analysis (perfusion = peak enhancement/area under arterial curve; see Chapter 4). In a group of 10 control subjects, Shih and Huang [38] found that the difference in peak attenuation between symmetrical brain regions of interest following a 50 ml bolus of 65% meglumine amidotrizoate was no more than 1.2 HU, equivalent to a relative difference of about 10–12%. This method of analysis also provides a straightforward way of producing functional images of relative cerebral perfusion.

Cerebral perfusion measurements are also possible using the gradient method of analysis (see Chapter 4). The functional images have high spatial resolution (Figure 6.10) but, unlike techniques using diffusible tracers, cerebral vessels are seen as areas of apparently high perfusion. This creates some difficulty in quantification as ROIs should avoid these areas if absolute perfusion values are required. Profiles drawn avoiding vessels, but including cortical grey matter and central white matter, give peak cortical values, of 0.7 ml/min/ml and trough white matter values of 0.2 ml/min/ml, close to values obtained with diffusible tracer methods [39].

SUMMARY

Perfusion CT offers a method for studying tissue perfusion with a number of advantages over other techniques. It is relatively non-invasive, requiring an intravenous injection only. Rather than provide relative perfusion values or perfusion indices, the technique can quantify perfusion in absolute units (i.e. ml/min/ml) with values close to those of other accepted techniques. The high spatial resolution enables small structures to be studied either with ROIs or with functional images. Even organs as small as the adrenals are potentially amenable to study (Figure 6.11). The high spatial resolution also allows regional variations in perfusion within organs, for example spleen and kidney, to be visualized directly rather than inferred from compartmental analysis. As perfusion CT can be performed on many existing CT systems, taking only a few minutes to perform, the technique could be readily adopted by X-ray departments throughout the world.

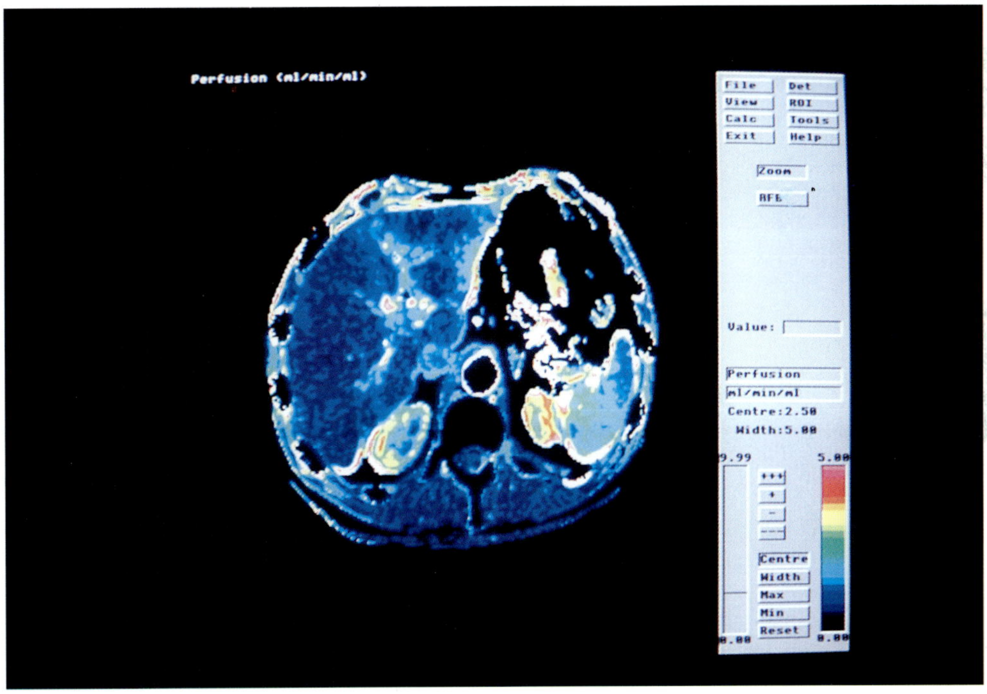

Figure 6.11
CT perfusion image of the upper abdomen including the left adrenal gland. Adrenal perfusion is measured at 1.5 ml/min/ml (pink: 5 ml/min/ml).

REFERENCES

1. Trueta, J., Barclay, A.E., Daniel, P.M. *et al.* (1947) Studies of the renal circulation. Oxford: Blackwell Scientific Publications.
2. Sherwood, T. and Lavender, J.P. (1971) Renal medulla perfusion. Direct observations by fine detail angiography in the dog. *Nephron*, **8**, 317–328.
3. Blaufox, M.D., Fromowitz, A., Gruskin A. *et al.* Validation of use of xenon-133 to measure intrarenal distribution of blood flow. *American Journal of Physiology*, **219**, 440–444.

4. Gruenewald, S.M., Nimmon, C.C., Nawaz, M.K. and Britton, K.E. (1981) A non-invasive γ-camera technique for the measurement of intrarenal flow distribution in man. *Clinical Science*, **61**, 385–389.
5. Ishikawa, I., Onouchi, Z., Saito, Y. *et al.* (1981) Renal cortex visualisation and analysis of dynamic CT curves of the kidney. *Journal of Computer Assisted Tomography* **5**, 695–701.
6. Probst, P., Mahler, F., Roesler, H. and Fuchs, W.A. (1983) Renal artery stenosis and evaluation of the effect of endoluminal dilatation: comparison of dynamic CT scanning and I-131-OIHA renogram. *Investigative Radiology*, **18**, 2664–2271.
7. Jansen, V.O., Gmelin, E., Burmester, E. *et al.* (1989) Analyse von dynamischen CT-kurven bei nierentransplantaten mit abstossungsreaktion und cyclosporin-A-intoxikation *ROFO*, **151**, 473–476.
8. Jaschke, W.R., Gould, R.G., Cogan, M.G., Sievers, R. and Lipton, M.J. (1987) Cine-CT measurement of cortical renal blood flow. *Journal of Computer Assisted Tomography*, **11**, 779–784.
9. Jaschke, W.R., Sievers, R., Lipton, M.J. and Cogan, M.G. (1989) Cine-computed tomographic assessment of regional renal blood flow. *Acta Radiologica*, **31**, 77–81.
10. Miles, K.A. (1991) Measurement of tissue perfusion by dynamic computed tomography. *British Journal of Radiology*, **64**, 409–412.
11. Miles, K.A., Hayball, M.P. and Dixon, A.K. (1994) Functional imaging of changes in human intrarenal perfusion using quantitative dynamic computed tomography. *Investigative Radiology*, **29**, 911–914.
12. Blomley, M.J.K., Kormano, M., Coulden, R. *et al.* (1994) Renal perfusion quantified with contrast enhanced CT. *Investigative Radiology*, **29**(2), S232–233.
13. Studley, J.G.N., Mathie, R.T. and Blumgart, L.H. (1987) Blood flow measurement in the canine pancreas. *Journal of Surgical Research*, **42**, 101–115.
14. Kubo, S., Yamamoto, K., Magata, Y., Iwaski, Y., Tamaki, N., Yonekura, Y. and Konishi, J. (1991) Assessment of pancreatic blood flow with positron emission tomography and oxygen-15 water. *Annals of Nuclear Medicine*, **51**, 133–138.
15. Miles, K.A., Hayball, M.P. and Dixon, A.K. (1995) Measurement of human pancreatic perfusion using dynamic computed tomography with perfusion imaging. *British Journal of Radiology*, **68**, 471–475.
16. Groom, A. (1987) Microcirculation of the spleen: new concepts, new challenges. *Microvascular Research*, **34**, 269–289.
17. Williams, R., Condon, R.E., Williams, H.S., Blendis, L.M. and Kreel, L. (1968) Splenic blood flow in cirrhosis and portal hypertension. *Clinical Science*, **34**, 441–452.
18. Gitlin, N., Grahame, G.R., Kreel, L., Williams, H.S. and Sherlock, S. (1970) Splenic blood flow and resistance in patients with cirrhosis before and after portacaval anastomoses. *Gastroenterology*, **59**, 208–213.
19. Ueda, H., Kitani, K., Kameda, H. *et al.* (1971) Splenic blood flow in idiopathic portal hypertension in Japan measured by 85-Kr clearance method. *Acta Hepato-splenology*, **18**, 28–40.
20. Huchzermeyer, H., Schmitz-Feuerhake, I. and Reblin, T. (1977) Determination of splenic blood flow by inhalation of radioactive rare gases. *European Journal of Clinical Investigation*, **7**, 345–349.
21. Takhasi, Y., Akasaka, K., Tanaka, Y., Syriyone, S. and Uyama, C. (1974) Studies on splenic blood flow and blood cell destruction by simulation analysis of radiosplenogram. *1st World Congress of Nuclear Medicine*, Tokyo, Kyoto pp. 97–101.

22. Blomley, M.J.K., Coulden, R.A., Lim-Dunham, J.E. *et al.* (1997) Splenic perfusion studied with UFCT. *Academic Radiology*, **4**, 13–20.
23. Miles, K.A., McPherson, S.J. and Hayball, M.P. (1995) Transient splenic inhomogeneity on contrast enhanced CT: mechanism and effect of liver disease. *Radiology*, **194**, 91–95.
24. Glazer, G.M., Axel, L., Goldberg, H.I. and Moss, A.A. (1981) Dynamic CT of the normal spleen. *American Journal of Roentgenology*, **137**, 343–346.
25. Ternberg, J.L. and Butcher, H.R. Jr. (1965) Blood-flow relation between hepatic artery and portal vein. *Science*, **150**, 1030–1031.
26. Ferguson, D.J. (1963) Haemodynamics in surgery for portal hypertension. *Annals of Surgery*, **158**, 383–386.
27. Sherriff, S.B., Smart, R.C. and Taylor, I. (1977) Clinical study of liver blood flow in man measured by ^{133}Xe clearance after portal vein injection. *Gut*, **18**, 1027.
28. Kashiwagi, T., Kimura, K., Suematsu, T. *et al.* (1981) Heterogeneous intrahepatic distribution of blood flow in humans. *European Journal of Nuclear Medicine*, **6**, 545–549.
29. Gates, G.F. and Dore, E.K. (1973) Streamline flow in the human portal vein. *Journal of Nuclear Medicine* **14**, 79–83.
30. Mathie, R.T. (1986) Hepatic blood flow measurement with inert gas clearance. *Journal of Surgical Research*, **41**, 92–110.
31. Miles, K.A., Hayball, M.P. and Dixon, A.K. (1993) Functional images of hepatic perfusion obtained with dynamic computed tomography. *Radiology*, **188**, 405–411.
32. Miles, K.A., Hayball, M.P. and Dixon, A.K. (1993) Quantitative dynamic computed tomography in the assessment of liver perfusion: differences between right and left lobes. *British Journal of Radiology*, (Congress Suppl) **66**, 103.
33. Blomley, M.J.K., Coulden, R. and Dawson, P. *et al.* (1995) Liver perfusion studied with ultrafast CT. *Journal of Computer Assisted Tomography*, **19**(3), 424–433.
34. Bonte, F.J., Devous, M.D. and Stokely, E.M. (1988) Tomographic imaging of regional cerebral blood flow with diffusible tracers. In *Diagnostic Nuclear Medicine* (eds A. Gottschalk, P.B. Hoffer, and E.J. Potchen), Vol. II, pp. 917–919. Baltimore: Williams & Wilkins.
35. Axel, L. (1980) Cerebral blood flow determination by rapid-sequence computed tomography; theoretical analysis. *Radiology*, **137**, 679–686.
36. Beringer, W.H., Axel, L., Norman, D., Napel, S. and Redington, R.W. (1981) Functional imaging of the brain using computed tomography. *Radiology*, **138**, 711–716.
37. Axel, L. (1983) Tissue mean transit time from dynamic computed tomography by a simple deconvolution technique. *Radiology*, **18**, 94–99.
38. Shih, T.T.F. and Huang, K-M. (1988) Acute stroke: detection of changes in cerebral perfusion with dynamic CT scanning. *Radiology*, **169**, 469–474.
39. Sinnatamby, R., Miles, K.A., Hayball, M.P. and Dixon, A.K. (1994) CT perfusion imaging of the brain: iodine or xenon? *British Journal of Radiology* (Congress Suppl), **67**, 135.

Chapter 7

APPLICATIONS OF PERFUSION CT

K. Miles and M. Blomley

To date, perfusion computed tomography (CT) has rarely formed part of the radiological assessment of patients in routine clinical practice. However, studies using this technique in various diseases have not only demonstrated the value of perfusion CT in research but have also revealed a number of potential clinical applications. As perfusion CT takes only a few minutes and can be performed on existing CT equipment, the technique could readily be incorporated into routine CT examinations in a number of clinical situations. This chapter considers the results and potential applications of perfusion CT in hepatology and nephrology (including transplantation), oncology, acute and chronic brain conditions and diseases of the pancreas. Cardiac imaging is covered in a separate chapter (Chapter 9). It is acknowledged by the authors that, due to the limited world experience with perfusion CT, this chapter should be seen as providing pointers to potential applications that need to be confirmed by wider experience.

HEPATOLOGY

Changes in hepatic perfusion in cirrhosis

CT evaluation of hepatic cirrhosis conventionally relies upon morphological features such as changes in the size, contour or homogeneity of the liver, the presence of ascites or varices and splenomegaly. However, there may be no detectable abnormality using such anatomical criteria, even in patients with proven cirrhosis. Furthermore, the correlation between disease severity and the degree of morphological change is poor.

Radionuclide studies can detect abnormalities of liver function resulting from cirrhosis before morphological changes are seen on CT. First-pass nuclear medicine techniques are used to determine the ratio of the arterial component to total liver blood flow (e.g. hepatic perfusion index, HPI). Increased values are found in cirrhosis and the degree of change correlates with disease severity [1,2]. The measurements can also be used to monitor changes with time and in response to therapeutic intervention.

On the other hand, nuclear medicine techniques lack specificity (for instance, the HPI is also raised in the presence of hepatic metastases). Perfusion CT can

Parameter	Normal controls Indirect	Normal controls Direct	Cirrhotics Indirect	Cirrhotics Direct
Arterial perfusion (ml/min/ml)	0.15	0.19	0.36	0.25
Portal perfusion (ml/min/ml)	0.34	0.93	0.17	0.43
Total perfusion (ml/min/ml)	0.50	1.12	0.59	0.68
Hepatic perfusion index (HPI)	0.32	0.17	0.65	0.37

* See also Chapter 6.

Table 7.1
Median values of perfusion in the right lobe of patients with cirrhosis and normal controls using either direct or indirect methods of determining portal perfusion*

combine the sensitivity of a functional evaluation with the specificity afforded by a morphological assessment.

Table 7.1 displays the changes in perfusion occurring in the right lobe of the liver in patients with proven hepatic cirrhosis as measured by perfusion CT. These data have been derived from two separate series using either the direct or indirect methods of measuring portal perfusion (see Chapter 6) [3,4]. As with nuclear medicine techniques, CT measurements of HPI, using either method, are increased in cirrhosis. CT has the added ability to evaluate portal and arterial perfusion separately. Thus, not only does CT demonstrate a reduction in portal perfusion (with direct and indirect methods), as would be expected in association with portal hypertension, but it also demonstrates an increase in arterial perfusion. This reflects the reciprocal relationship between the two circulations of the liver whereby a reduction in flow within one system is associated with an increase in the other (see Chapter 6). Measurements of combined arterial and direct portal perfusion are reduced in cirrhosis, in keeping with the results of

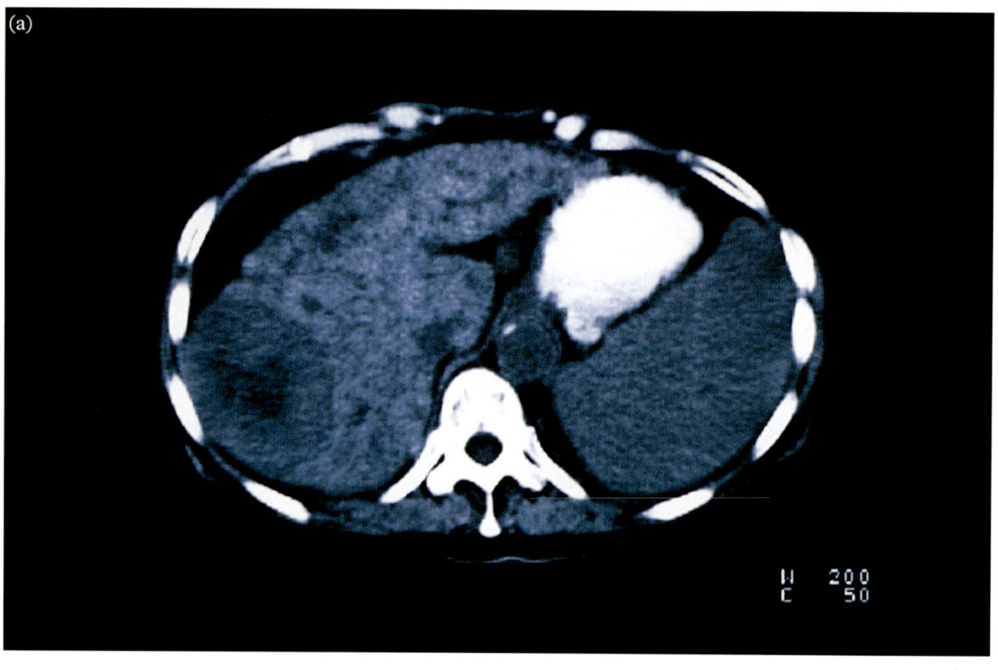

Figure 7.1
(a) Conventional CT, (b) arterial perfusion image. (c) indirect portal perfusion in a patient with hepatic cirrhosis and a hepatocellular carcinoma in the right lobe. The tumour demonstrates high arterial perfusion. Portal perfusion is reduced in the remaining liver, reflecting portal hypertension.

Figure 7.1
(*continued*)

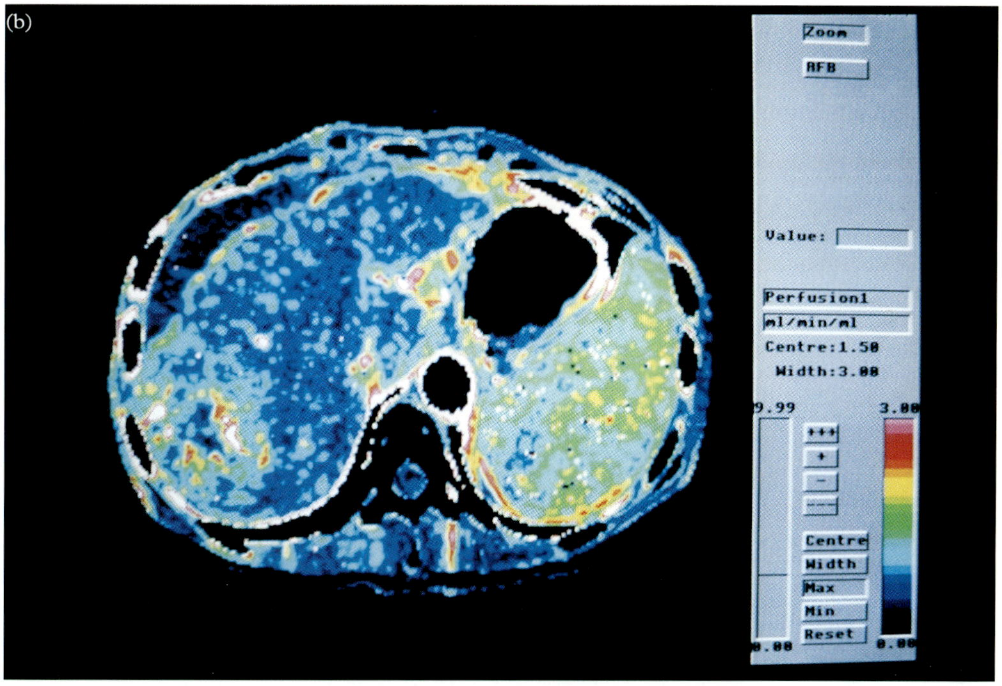

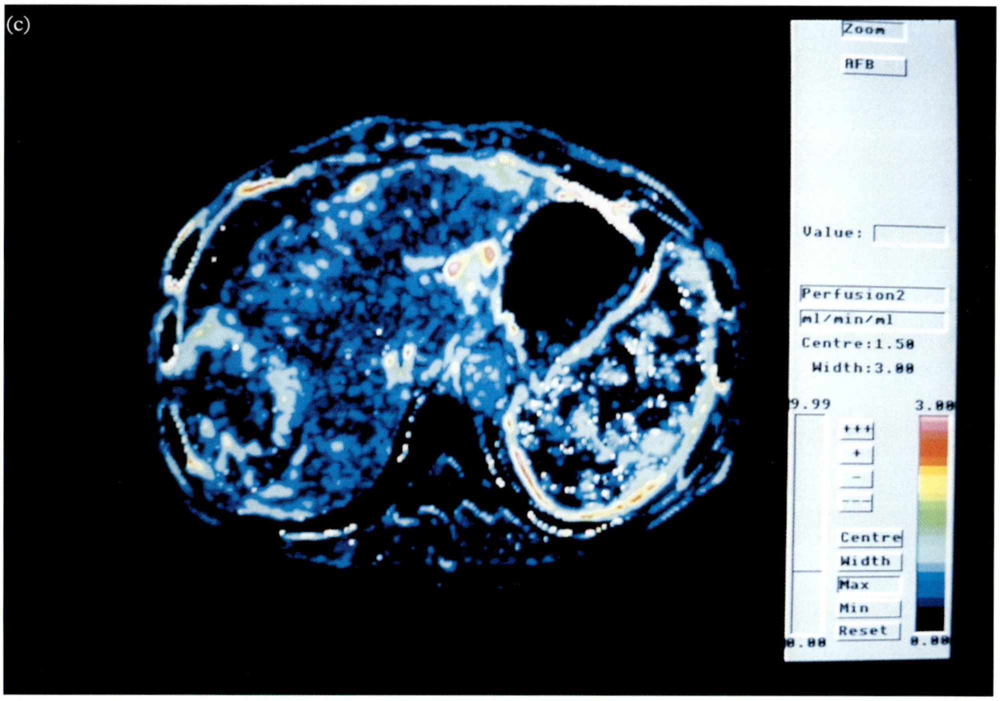

inert gas wash-out studies. This is not seen when using the indirect technique, probably due to the underestimation of portal perfusion that occurs when using this method; the underestimated fall in portal perfusion is swamped by the more accurately measured increase in arterial perfusion.

The transaxial format of perfusion CT images also allows measurement of differential changes in the left lobe (Figure 7.1). This has not been possible with first-pass nuclear medicine techniques due to the inclusion of a vascular signal

Table 7.2
Hepatic perfusion values: ratios of right to left lobes

Parameter	Normal controls	Cirrhotics
Arterial perfusion (ml/min/ml)	0.71	0.78
Portal perfusion (ml/min/ml) (indirect method)	1.27	0.55
Total perfusion (ml/min/ml)	0.89	0.74
Hepatic perfusion index (HPI)	0.58	1.43

within a left lobe region of interest (ROI) due to the close proximity of heart and great vessels. Using perfusion CT, cirrhosis can be seen to affect the haemodynamics within right and left lobes differently (Table 7.2). For arterial perfusion, the ratio between the lobes is similar for controls and patients with cirrhosis, with higher values seen in the left lobe. However, the trend for higher portal perfusion in the right lobe, seen in the normal liver, is reversed in cirrhosis. This relative preservation of portal perfusion within the left lobe is in keeping with greater total perfusion seen in the left lobe in cirrhosis using inert-gas wash-out techniques [5]. It may also be related to the phenomenon of left-lobe hypertrophy seen in cirrhosis as liver mass is thought to be dependent on portal and not arterial blood flow, a fact demonstrable following partial liver resection [6].

Changes in splenic perfusion in hepatic cirrhosis

Changes in global and regional splenic perfusion also occur in patients with hepatic cirrhosis. Although splenic blood flow is usually increased in cirrhosis, this largely results from enlargement of the organ. Perfusion (i.e. blood flow per unit volume) is reduced, however. This has been observed with inert-gas wash-out techniques but can also be seen with perfusion CT [9,10]. Similar results have been found when using either the gradient or Mullani–Gould methods of analysis (see Chapter 4). Normal values of 1.40 ml/min/ml and 1.29 ml/min/ml, are found using gradient and Mullani–Gould methods, respectively, compared with 1.13 ml/min/ml and 0.87 ml/min/ml in patients with cirrhosis.

Perfusion CT is unique in allowing direct visualization and measurement of regional changes in splenic perfusion in hepatic cirrhosis. Using the techniques outlined in Chapter 5, it has been possible to quantify the changes in perfusion in the fast- and slow-transit pathways of the splenic microcirculation and to observe shifts in the relative sizes of the two pathways. The perfusion (gradient method) and sizes of the two pathways from a study comparing normal and cirrhotic subjects [9] are given in Table 7.3.

Although perfusion falls in both pathways, the decrease is greater in the slow pathway. There is also an increase in the relative size of the slow pathway. These characteristic changes can also be seen with perfusion imaging as well as ROI analysis. Transient splenic homogeneity is a normal finding on dynamic CT,

Table 7.3
Changes in splenic perfusion with hepatic cirrhosis

Parameter	Controls	Cirrhotics
Fast pathway perfusion (ml/min/ml)	1.44	1.22
Relative size of fast pathway (%)	77	65
Slow pathway perfusion (ml/min/ml)	1.24	0.89
Relative size of slow pathway (%)	23	35
Global splenic perfusion (ml/min/ml)	1.40	1.13

reflecting the two perfusion pathways, but the findings from dynamic splenic CT suggest this phenomenon will be marked in patients with cirrhosis. The slow pathway corresponds to the red pulp where red cells are conditioned prior to destruction. The finding of an increase in the size of this pathway also provides a mechanism for the hypersplenism that occurs in some patients with hepatic cirrhosis.

The above study found that a global splenic perfusion of less than 1 ml/min/ml only occurred in cirrhosis. It also suggested that measurements of perfusion in the slow-transit pathway may be a highly sensitive method for detecting portal hypertension non-invasively. Reduced slow-pathway perfusion was found even in patients with normal portal vein blood velocities on examination with Doppler ultrasound.

Liver transplantation

A competent vascular supply allowing adequate tissue perfusion is vital to the survival of any transplanted organ. Clearly, if perfusion falls below a certain threshold, then tissue infarction will occur. Less severe ischaemia has been implicated as a possible aetiological factor in biliary anastomotic failure and possibly chronic rejection of liver allografts. With liver allografts, the situation is complicated by the dual blood supply, arterial and portal, to this organ and primary vascular complications can occur in either system. Changes in allograft perfusion may also be secondary to pathological processes occurring within the transplanted organ itself.

The supply of blood to the transplanted liver can be evaluated in a number of ways. Deteriorating organ function due to ischaemia may be first suggested by changes in blood biochemistry but elucidation of the underlying cause frequently relies upon imaging. Angiography provides detailed anatomical information with a subjective assessment of blood flow but is invasive. Doppler ultrasound is

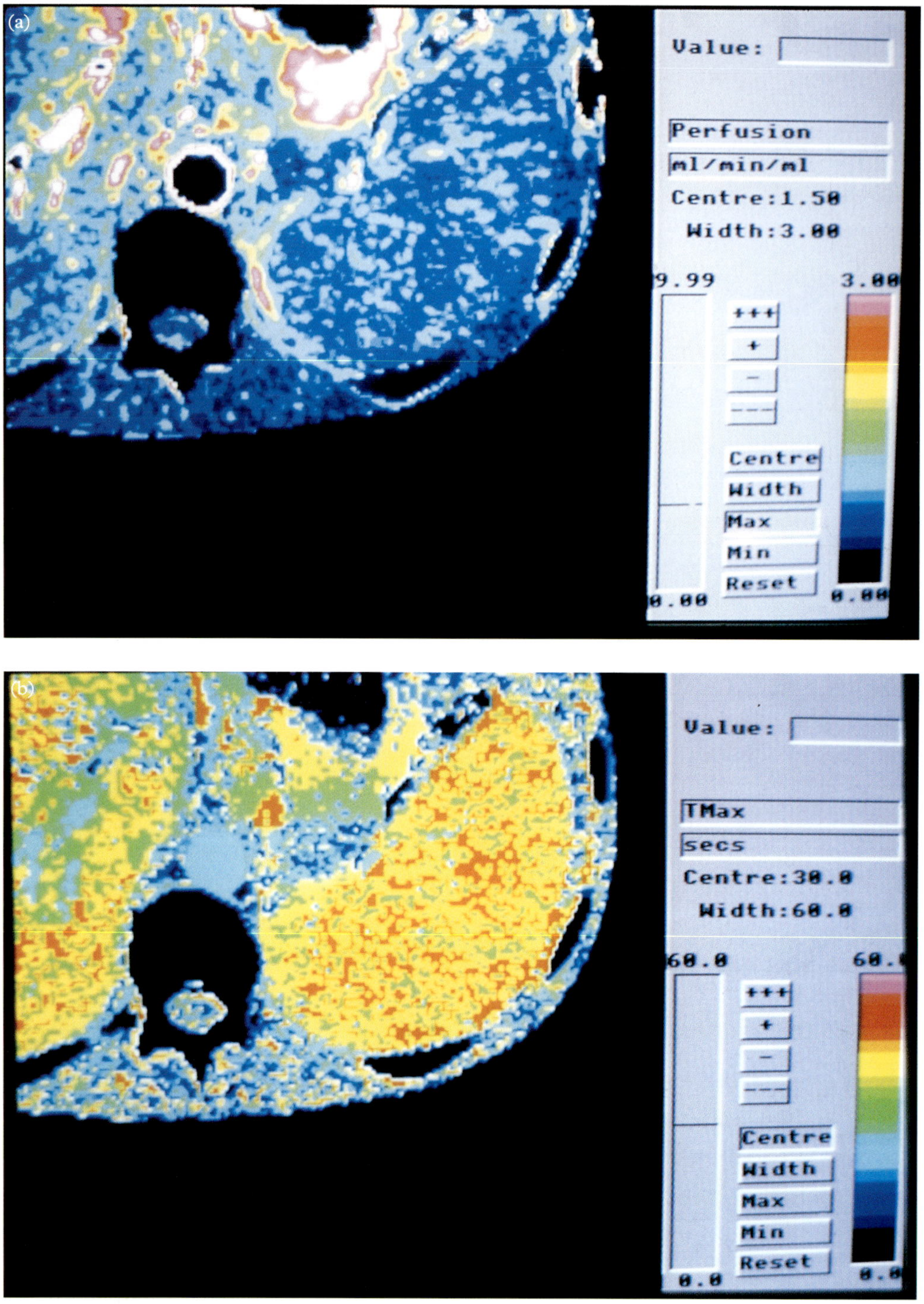

Figure 7.2
(a) Perfusion and (b) time to maximum enhancement images of the spleen in a patient with hepatic cirrhosis (blue: low perfusion/early enhancement; red: high perfusion [3 ml/min/ml]/late enhancement). Note the greater part of the spleen enhances late. Perfusion is low in both pathways (cf. Figure 6.6, page 78).

widely used to good effect but evaluation of regional changes within an organ is generally limited to segmental vessels and does not assess capillary perfusion. Colloid scintigraphy has also been used and, although providing an evaluation of tissue perfusion, is constrained by poor spatial resolution. Ultimately, biopsy of the allograft may be required but is not without potential complications.

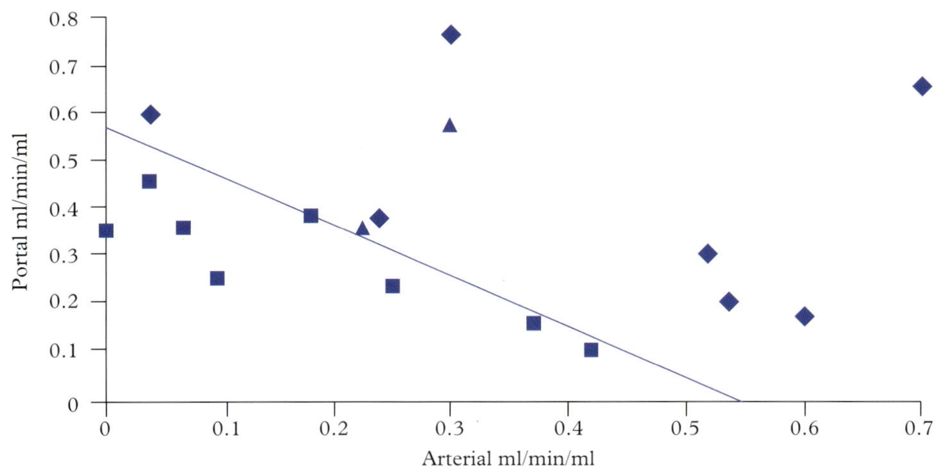

Figure 7.3
Right lobe arterial and (indirect) portal perfusion values from failed and successful liver allografts. An apparent threshold of 0.55 ml/min/ml for combined arterial and portal perfusion is indicated. ■ = Failed; ▲ = equivocal; ◆ = successful

As yet, perfusion CT is not routinely used in the evaluation of liver allografts but the results of research demonstrate the potential of the technique in this area. By evaluating arterial and portal perfusion at the capillary level, the functional effects of primarily vascular disease (e.g. thrombosis) upon perfusion within the tissues distally can be assessed and pathological processes arising within the transplanted organ, but with associated perfusion changes, are detectable. The spatial resolution of functional CT enables regional changes in perfusion to be determined. The absolute quantification allows allograft perfusion to be assessed with respect to ischaemic thresholds.

Figure 7.3 plots right-lobe arterial and portal perfusion from a number of patients with successful and failed liver allografts [11]. Amongst the successful grafts, a great variability in arterial and portal perfusion is seen. The reciprocal relationship between the two circulations is preserved in the transplanted liver as in some cases low arterial perfusion appears to be compensated by high portal perfusion and vice versa. The data suggest that combined arterial and portal perfusion is a more critical parameter. All transplants with combined values below 0.55 ml/min/ml demonstrated a poor outcome suggesting an ischaemic threshold which is close to values found in the normal liver.

The functional effects of vascular complications upon hepatic perfusion can be evaluated. For instance, the presence of adequate collateral vessels in the presence of a lobar arterial stenosis or occlusion can be confirmed (Figure 7.4). Similarly, the functional significance of portal vein thrombosis can be evaluated by confirming the presence of a satisfactory compensatory increase in arterial perfusion with maintenance of total perfusion above the critical threshold (Figure 7.5).

Chronic rejection of liver allografts is associated with reduced perfusion (Figure 7.6). The pathological changes of rejection are said to start centrally within the liver and thus percutaneous biopsy of the liver periphery may miss the diagnosis in the early stages. There is anecdotal evidence that demonstration of the perfusion changes in rejection has the potential to make the diagnosis earlier.

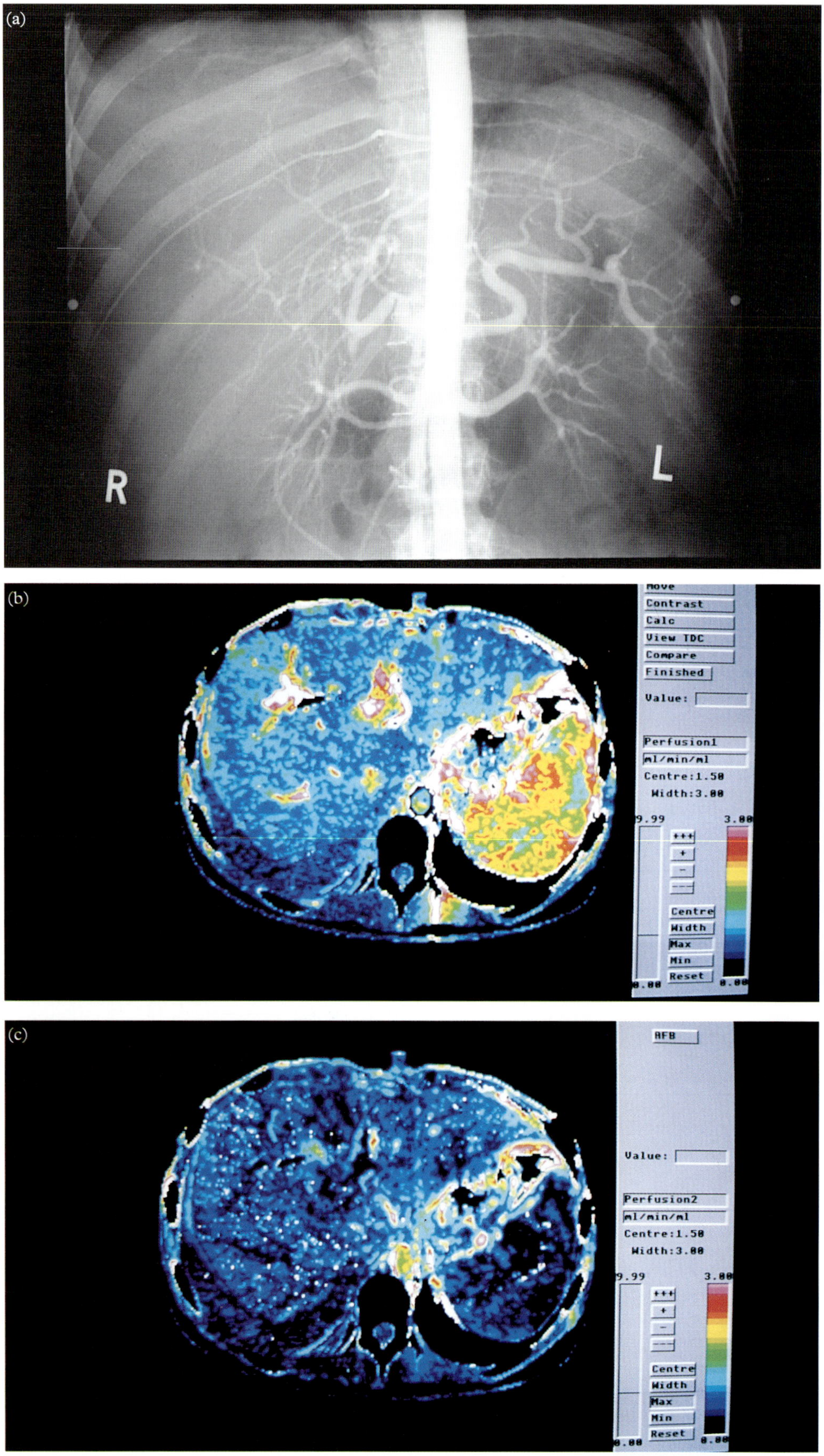

Figure 7.4
A hepatic angiogram (a) and CT perfusion images (b) arterial; (c) indirect portal; pink = 3 ml/min/ml) in a liver-transplant recipient with an occluded right hepatic artery. Perfusion images confirm adequate perfusion despite the arterial occlusion. The allograft survived.

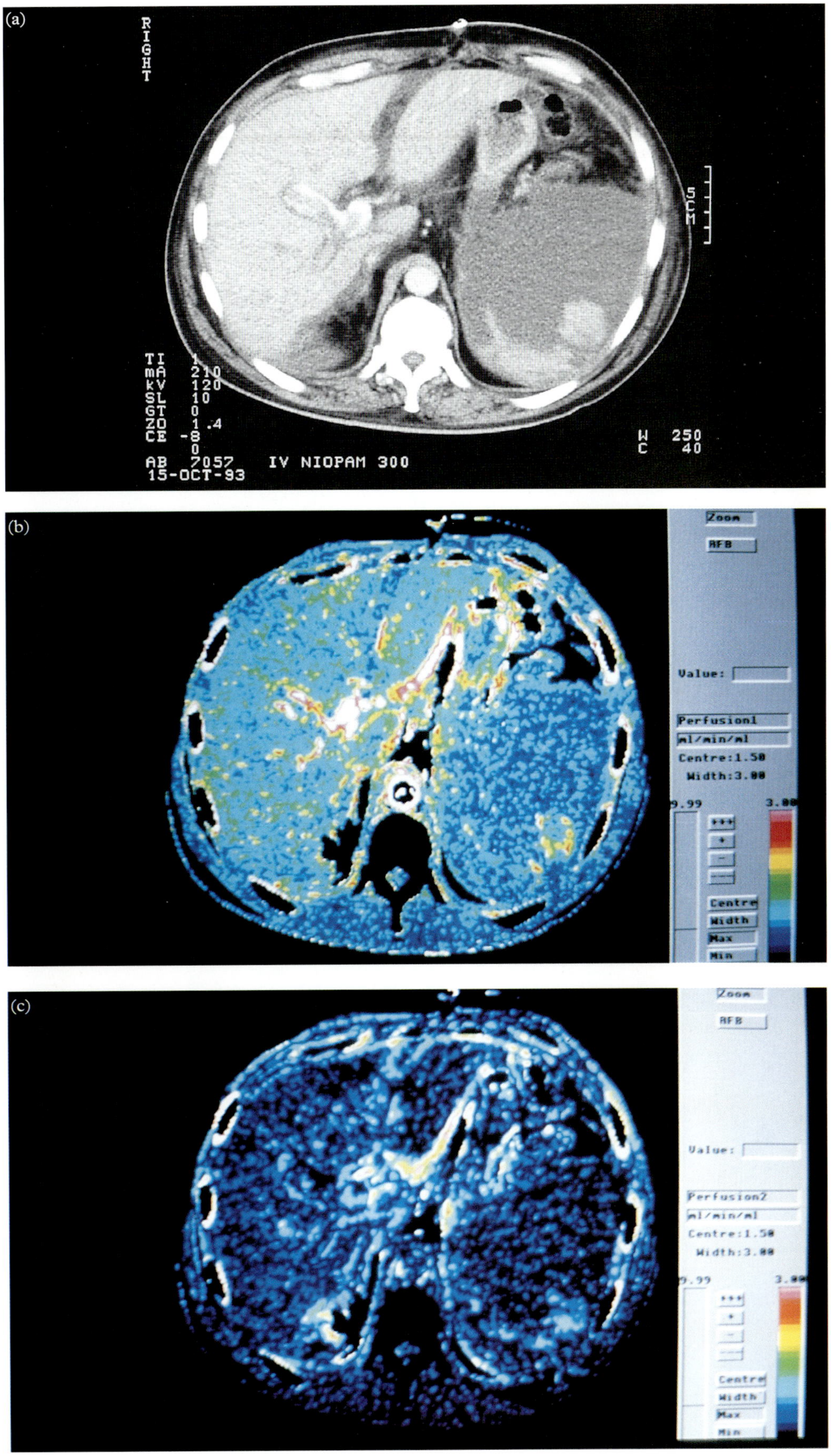

Figure 7.5
The conventional contrast enhanced CT (a) demonstrates portal vein thrombosis in a liver-transplant recipient. The arterial perfusion image (b) demonstrates increased arterial perfusion values which compensate for the reduced portal perfusion (c) (pink = 3 ml/min/ml).

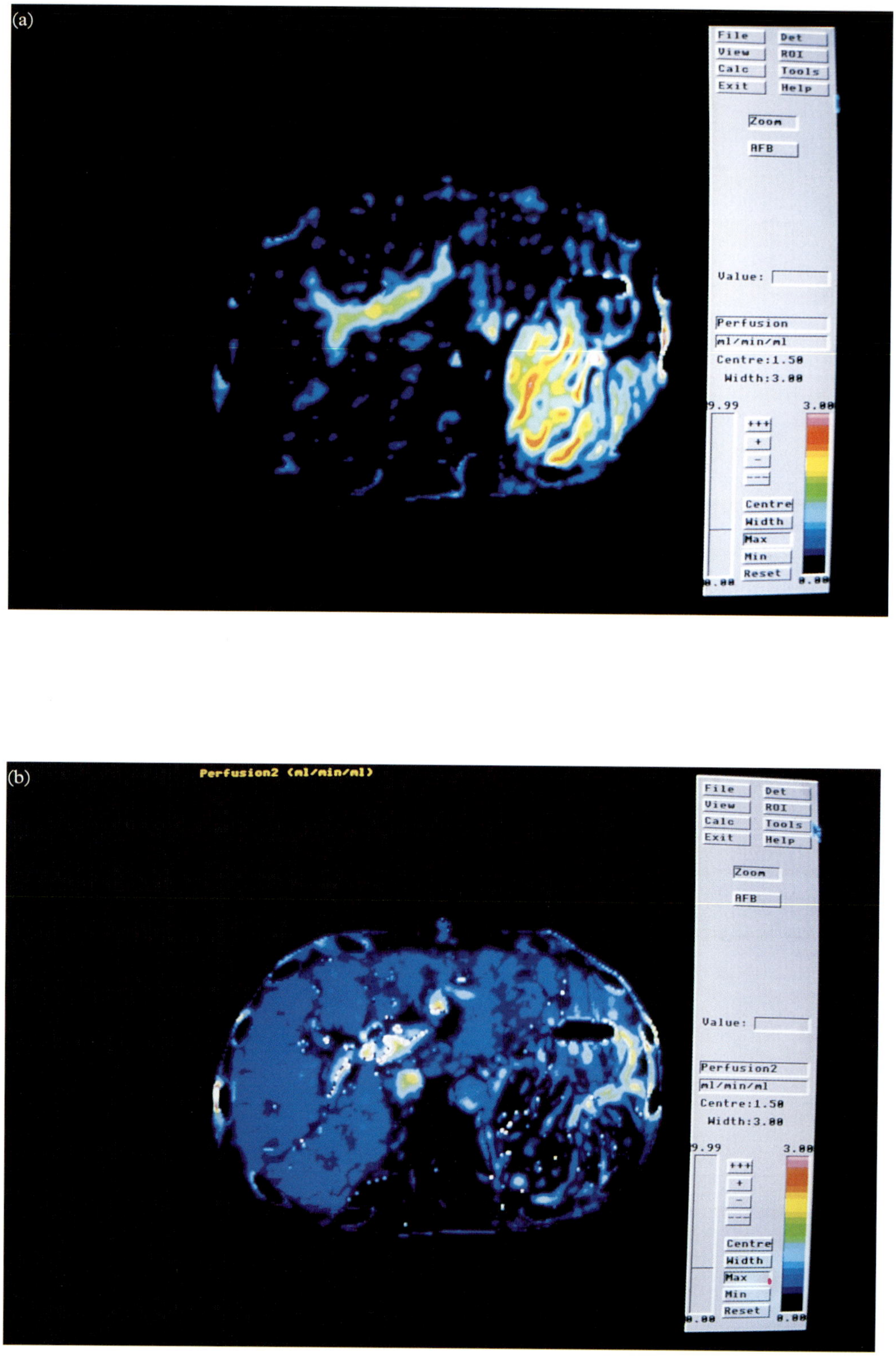

Figure 7.6
Arterial (a) and (indirect) portal (b) perfusion images of a liver transplant undergoing rejection (pink: 3 ml/min/ml). Arterial perfusion is virtually absent with low–moderate portal perfusion. Retransplantation was subsequently required.

Other liver diseases

Changes in hepatic perfusion have also been observed with focal liver lesions and are discussed in the oncology section below.

NEPHROLOGY

Changes in kidney blood flow have been demonstrated in a variety of renal diseases using techniques such as isotope renography and Doppler ultrasound. Only perfusion CT, however, offers the ability to measure absolute perfusion in different areas of the kidney and thus, for example, allow direct measurement of differential cortical and medullary perfusion. This provides an opportunity to further categorize renal diseases on account of changes in the intrarenal distribution of blood flow due to differing effects upon cortical and medullary perfusion measured separately. Not only is the technique applicable to renal disease in general but also to renal allografts and in patients on cyclosporin following transplantation of other organs.

Hypertension

Analysis of renal time–attenuation curves has been used to assess patients with renal artery stenosis before and after angioplasty [12,13]. Although changes in perfusion parameters were observed, in general, assessment of renal transit by measuring the time taken for renal and cortical time–density curves to cross proved more helpful. Heinz *et al.* [14] demonstrated a reduced gradient in the cortical time–density curve in ischaemic canine kidneys. Probst *et al.* [12] measured the difference in peak enhancement between the two kidneys in controls and patients with renal artery stenosis. From the Mullani–Gould equation (Chapter 4), this can be considered a measure of relative perfusion. A significant difference in peak enhancement of 16 HU was reversed when angioplasty was successful but unchanged when there had been no response or partial improvement.

Although underestimating cortical perfusion, due to poor temporal resolution of the CT system used, Miles [15] demonstrated a selective reduction in cortical perfusion with normal medullary perfusion in patients with hypertension without renal artery stenosis. These changes were reversed following administration of the angiotensin-converting enzyme (ACE), inhibitor, captopril (Table 7.4). Overall, the findings were in accordance with those of Grunewald *et al.* [16] who used deconvolutional analysis of isotope renograms.

Perfusion CT of the kidneys can be a useful adjunct to spiral CT assessment of abdominal aortic aneurysms [17]. To ensure optimal timing of the contrast-enhanced spiral acquisition, it is accepted practice to perform an initial single-level dynamic sequence with a small bolus of contrast medium. This initial sequence can be exploited to simultaneously obtain information on perfusion without additional cost or radiation burden. Low pre-operative renal cortical perfusion predicts greater renal impairment following surgery, even with infrarenal aneurysms [17].

Table 7.4
Mean perfusion values for renal cortex and medulla in controls, patients with renal failure and hypertensives with and without captopril*

Patients	Cortical perfusion (ml/min/ml)	Medullary perfusion (ml/min/ml)
Control subjects	2.5	1.1
Renal failure	1.7	0.5
Hypertension without ACE inhibitor**	1.2	0.9
Hypertension with ACE inhibitor**	2.2	1.0

* In this study, cortical perfusion is underestimated due to poor temporal resolution of earlier CT systems but the differing effects on cortex and medulla are shown.
** ACE = angiotensin-converting enzyme.

It should be noted that, when measuring perfusion with CT, an error will be introduced if there is an arterial stenosis between the artery used for determining the input function for the calculation and the tissue of interest. This situation applies when measuring renal cortical perfusion in cases of renal artery stenosis. The presence of a stenosis will alter the geometry of the contrast medium bolus. The bolus shape distal to the stenosis, i.e. the true input for the renal cortex, is different from the input function that is actually measured proximal to the stenosis. This will result in the measured perfusion being lower than actual values. However, this may not matter clinically as the apparent value will still reflect the severity of the stenosis.

Renal failure

The time taken for aortic and cortical time–density curves (cortico-aortic time) to cross has been proposed as a semiquantitative measure of cortical perfusion in patients with acute tubular necrosis [18]. This time was found to be prolonged (>180 s) in the anuric phase, whereas a time of less than 180 s heralded the onset of diuresis. However, this index does not truly measure perfusion and will also be affected by filtration.

Absolute perfusion measurements show that renal failure is commonly associated with a reduction both in cortical and medullary perfusion (Table 7.4). In the dog, prerenal causes of renal failure, such as hypotension, have been reported to be associated with reduced cortical and medullary perfusion in some cases [19] although medullary perfusion is preserved in others [20]. In man, renal and obstructive causes of renal failure are associated with reduced cortical and medullary perfusion, a pattern distinct from that found in hypertensive subjects [15]. Single-location dynamic sequences at the level of the renal vein have been proposed to evaluate vascular invasion from renal carcinoma. Such a protocol can also be used simultaneously to evaluate renal perfusion and may usefully reveal unsuspected contralateral renal disease prior to nephrectomy [21].

Renal transplantation

Although not strictly evaluating perfusion alone, the cortico-aortic time has also been proposed as a method of assessing the physiological status of renal transplants [22]. Values are increased in allografts that are undergoing rejection when compared to normally functioning transplants. Although there was some overlap between the groups, the authors proposed that values above 60 s implied rejection. The corticomedullary time, however, provided better discrimination.

Jansen *et al.* [23] evaluated perfusion using the cortico-aortic time as well as the cortex/aorta and medulla/aorta slopes ratios. The results are summarized in Table 7.5. Acute tubular necrosis could be distinguished from rejection and cyclosporin toxicity as medullary perfusion was preserved with only a mild reduction in cortical perfusion. The authors also suggested that cyclosporin toxicity could be distinguished from rejection on the grounds that the former demonstrated a more marked reduction in cortical perfusion. Both pathologies were associated with reduced perfusion within the medulla.

Table 7.5
Perfusion changes in renal allografts (from Jansen *et al.* [23])

Patients	Cortico-aortic time (s)	Cortex/aorta slopes ratio	Medulla/aorta slopes ratio
Normal function	31	0.82	0.40
Acute tubular necrosis	31	0.72	0.36
Rejection	43	0.59	0.20
Cyclosporin toxicity	66	0.42	0.18

CT perfusion imaging has also been successfully applied to renal transplants, although experience is limited [24]. The technique was able to confirm allograft infarction (Figure 7.7) and has also demonstrated reduced cortical and medullary perfusion in an allograft with acute cellular rejection and tubular necrosis (Figure 7.8).

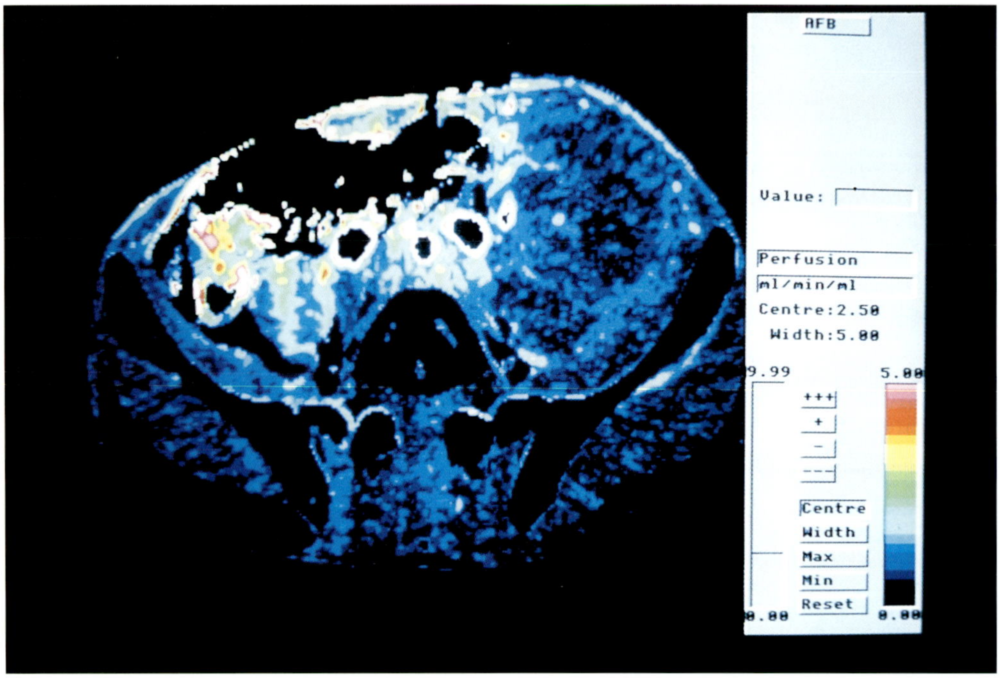

Figure 7.7
CT perfusion image demonstrating infarction of a renal allograft in the left iliac fossa (pink: 5 ml/min/ml) (cf. normal kidney, Figure 6.2, page 73).

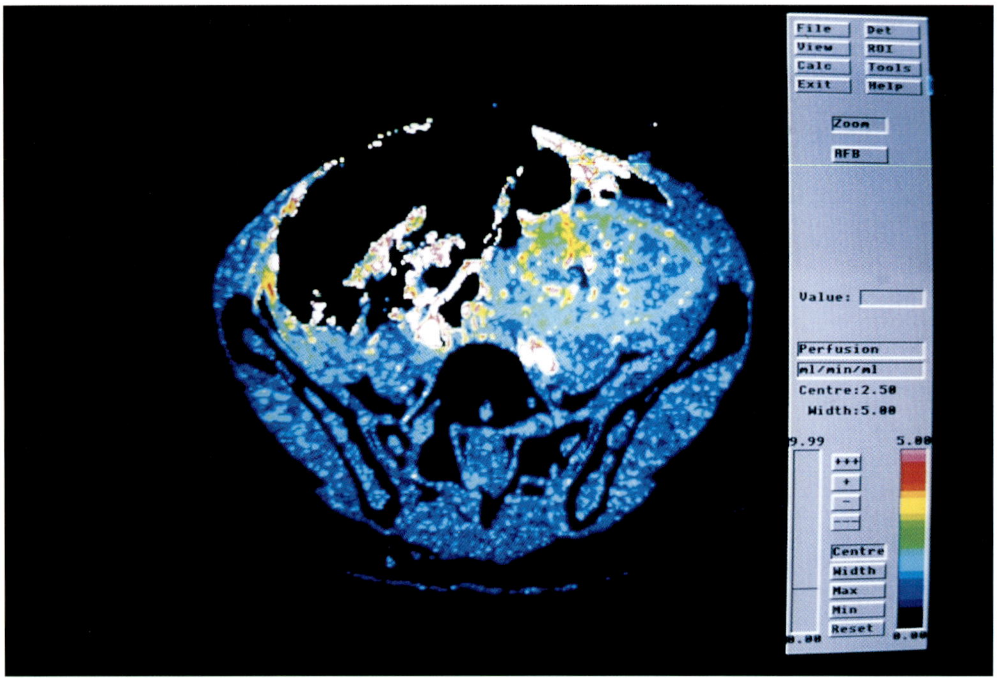

Figure 7.8
CT perfusion image of a renal transplant undergoing acute cellular rejection and tubular necrosis (pink: 5 ml/min/ml; cf. normal kidney, Figure 6.2, page 73).

Cyclosporin toxicity in native kidneys

The renal toxicity of cyclosporin is also of concern to recipients of other transplanted organs, including heart and liver. Compared with renal transplant recipients, evaluation of renal perfusion in these patients is less likely to be complicated by other pathological processes affecting perfusion. More recent experience of studying cyclosporin toxicity in liver transplant recipients [11,24] demonstrates reduced cortical and medullary perfusion (Figures 7.9 and 7.10) in keeping with the findings of Jansen *et al.* [23] in transplanted kidneys. However, in milder cases, medullary perfusion may be only slightly affected (Table 7.5). The severity of the toxicity also correlates with the degree of reduction in cortical perfusion.

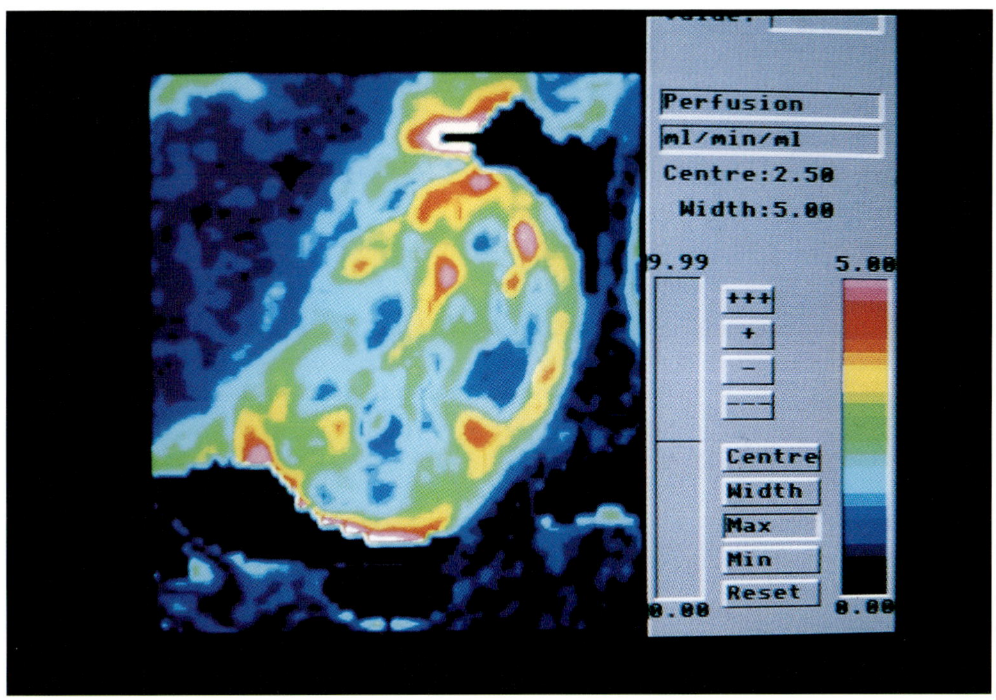

Figure 7.9
CT perfusion image of a kidney in a liver transplant recipient with renal cyclosporin toxicity (pink: 5 ml/min/ml; cf. normal kidney, Figure 6.2, page 73).

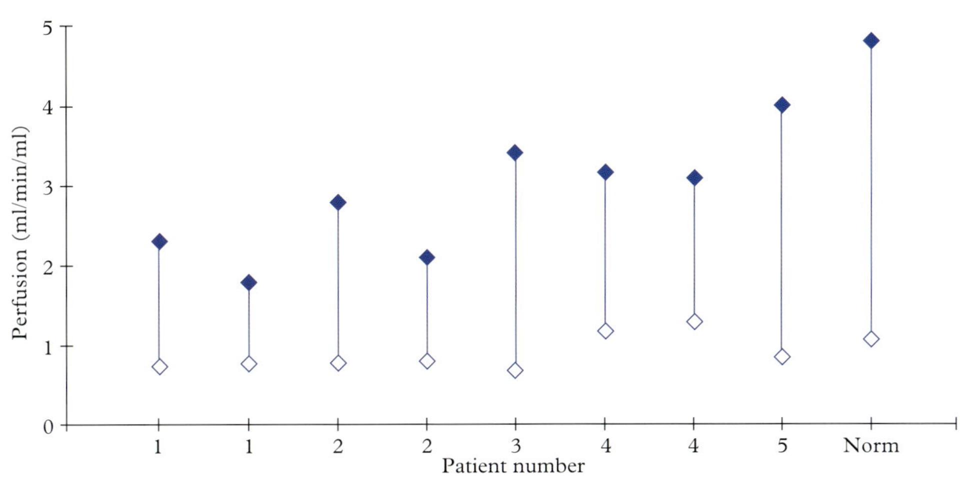

Figure 7.10
Renal cortical and medullary perfusion values in liver transplant recipients arranged by severity of cyclosporin effect. Blood levels are highest in patients on the left. Normal perfusion values are shown on the right. ◆ = cortex; ◇ = medulla (R. Sinnatamby, personal communication).

ONCOLOGY

The imaging of cancer is of increasing importance due to the greater prevalence of tumours in an ageing population and the success of cancer therapy resulting in increased numbers of survivors and a need to monitor the therapeutic response. To date, CT diagnostic criteria have largely relied upon morphological features such as the presence or change in size of a mass. However, such an approach cannot detect tumours within small lymph nodes and may not distinguish post-therapy fibrosis from active tumour.

Tumours display increased numbers of abnormal blood vessels, reflecting tumour neo-angiogenesis, and in general the active portion of malignant tumours exhibit increased perfusion. Indeed, there is evidence largely from nuclear medicine techniques, but also X-ray angiography and Doppler ultrasound, that perfusion can be used as a marker of tumour viability. Tumour perfusion is also more heterogeneous than normal tissues. The zone of neo-angiogenesis is located peripherally and has high perfusion whilst the tumour centre frequently becomes poorly perfused and necrotic as the mass ‘outgrows’ its blood supply. The source of blood supply may also differ between tumours and normal tissues. For example, unlike the surrounding liver, hepatic metastases derive their perfusion almost exclusively from the hepatic arterial system. Many patients with cancer already undergo CT and the simple inclusion of a perfusion sequence into existing conventional CT protocols would allow the differences in perfusion and microcirculation between normal and malignant tissues to be exploited. Such a combined structural and functional approach could potentially improve the sensitivity and specificity of CT in the detection of malignancy.

CT measurements of tumour perfusion have been shown to correlate well with the results of thermal clearance and positron emission tomography (PET) techniques [25] and generally, but not consistently, demonstrate increased values in tumours as compared with normal tissues (Table 7.6). The high spatial resolution of CT perfusion images enables direct visualization of the heterogeneous nature of tumour perfusion. High perfusion is seen peripherally with reduced values centrally (Figure 7.11) corresponding to the zone of angiogenesis surrounding central necrosis, as described above. In some instances, benign lesions exhibit higher perfusion than malignancies. For instance, pancreatic islet-cell tumours demonstrate a greater peak rate of enhancement than adenocarcinomas [26] and focal nodular hyperplasia typically has higher perfusion than hepatocellular carcinoma or hepatic metastases [27]. Thus, perfusion measurements can afford a degree of tissue characterization (Figure 7.12).

Tumours may also manifest functional effects upon surrounding tissues or distant organs, including effects on perfusion. This is of particular interest in the liver. Figure 7.13 plots arterial and portal perfusion values in the liver immediately adjacent to a mass and compares them to normal perfusion values. The perfusion of the adjacent liver is clearly abnormal in all cases. Arterial perfusion in the adjacent liver is increased whereas the effect on portal perfusion is more varied. There are a number of possible reasons for this. In some instances, increased pressure within a liver segment may reduce portal perfusion

Table 7.6
CT-perfusion values from various tumours compared with normal tissues and some benign lesions

Organ	Tissue	Cases (n)	Perfusion (ml/min/ml)
Kidney	Normal cortex	14	4.7
	Renal carcinoma	2	5.1
Liver	Normal arterial	5	0.17
	Hepatocellular carcinoma	2	0.65
	Metastases	5	0.95
	Focal nodular hyperplasia	8	1.36
	Focal fat	1	0.10
Brain	Normal grey matter	9	0.7
	Normal white matter	9	0.2
	Glioma	1	0.5
	Meningioma	1	1.2

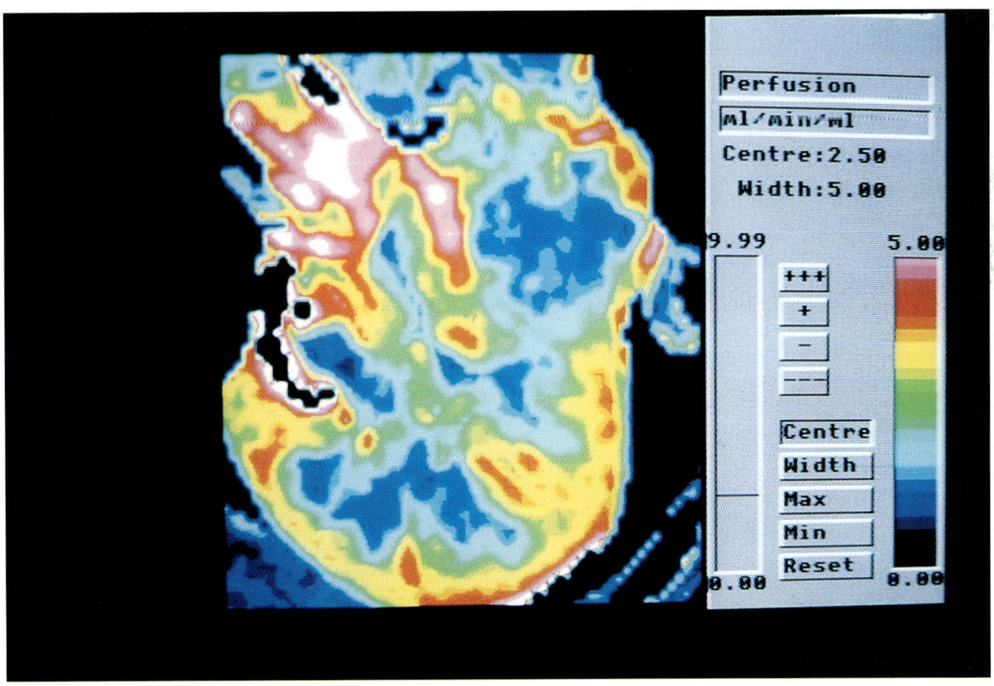

Figure 7.11
CT perfusion image of a renal carcinoma showing high peripheral perfusion and lower perfusion centrally (pink: 5 ml/min/ml).

with a reflex increase in arterial perfusion. Alternatively, the highly perfused metastases may produce a steal effect or a vasoactive humoral factor may be released by the primary tumour or metastasis.

Such a humoral mechanism has been proposed as an explanation for the finding of raised arterial perfusion in patients with colonic cancer but no overt

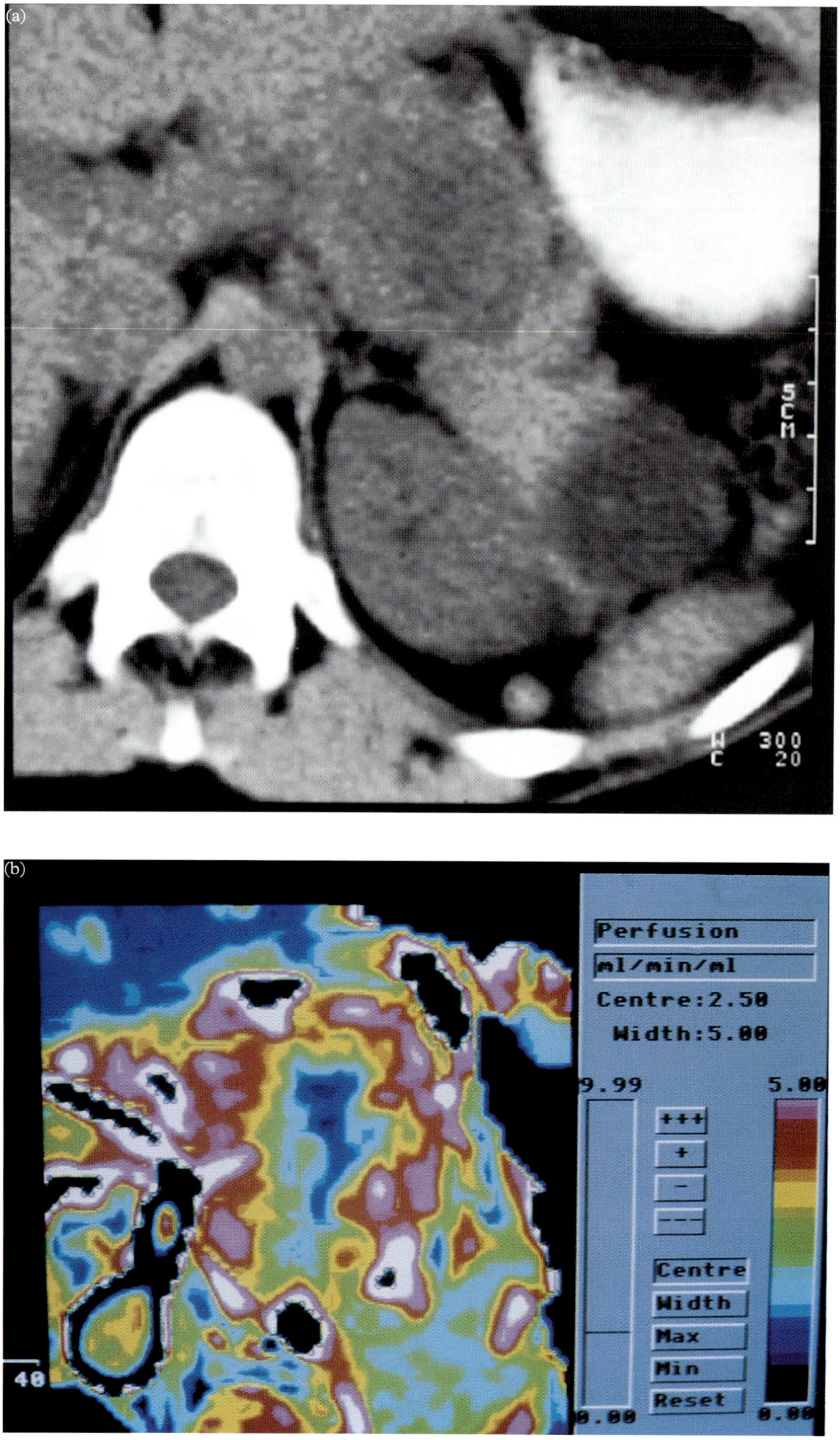

Figure 7.12
(a) Conventional CT and (b) perfusion image of a pancreatic islet-cell tumour. Note the high peripheral perfusion with lower values centrally (pink: 5 ml/min/ml).

Figure 7.13
Arterial and portal perfusion in liver tissue *surrounding* metastases as compared with normal values. Note that perfusion is abnormal adjacent to metastases. ◆ = metastasis; ☐ = normal.

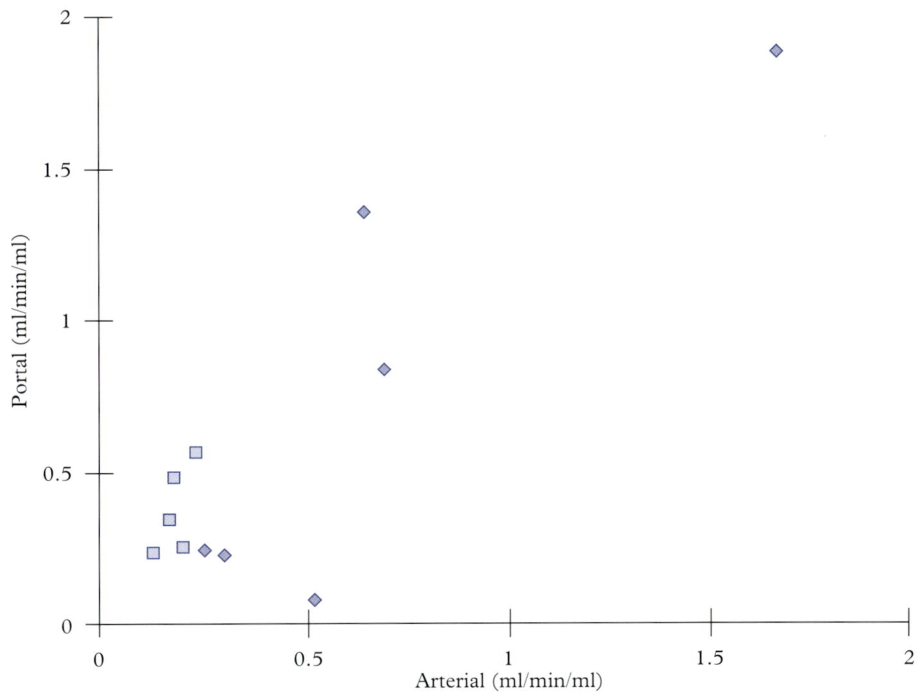

metastases [28]. These patients are significantly more likely to develop frank metastases within one year than those with normal liver perfusion. Inclusion of CT perfusion imaging within the conventional CT assessment of patients with colorectal cancer offers the potential of identifying those patients with a poorer outcome for whom adjuvant chemotherapy may be of particular benefit.

Whatever the mechanism, this finding has implications for protocols for conventional contrast-enhanced imaging of the liver as it is the hepatic perfusion that determines the delivery of contrast agents to the liver. This is particularly so since the advent of modern spiral CT equipment as the radiologist now has the choice of imaging within either the arterial or portal phase of enhancement. Firstly, it can be seen that studies on the enhancement patterns of normal livers do not provide a satisfactory model for hepatic enhancement in the presence of metastases. Liver metastases derive their blood supply almost exclusively from the arterial circulation. This can be seen on CT perfusion images in which metastases tend to demonstrate increased arterial perfusion but with markedly reduced portal perfusion (Figure 7.14). As the adjacent liver also has increased arterial perfusion, there will be no benefit in lesion-to-tissue contrast by imaging within the arterial phase of liver enhancement. On the other hand, as the adjacent liver may demonstrate normal or increased portal perfusion, whereas metastases have decreased portal perfusion, there will be improved lesion-to-tissue contrast in the portal phase.

In the context of detecting hepatocellular carcinomas on the background of hepatic cirrhosis, the situation becomes even more complicated due to the effects of cirrhosis on liver perfusion. As with metastases, the tumour demonstrates increased arterial perfusion but so does the cirrhotic liver. The tumour also

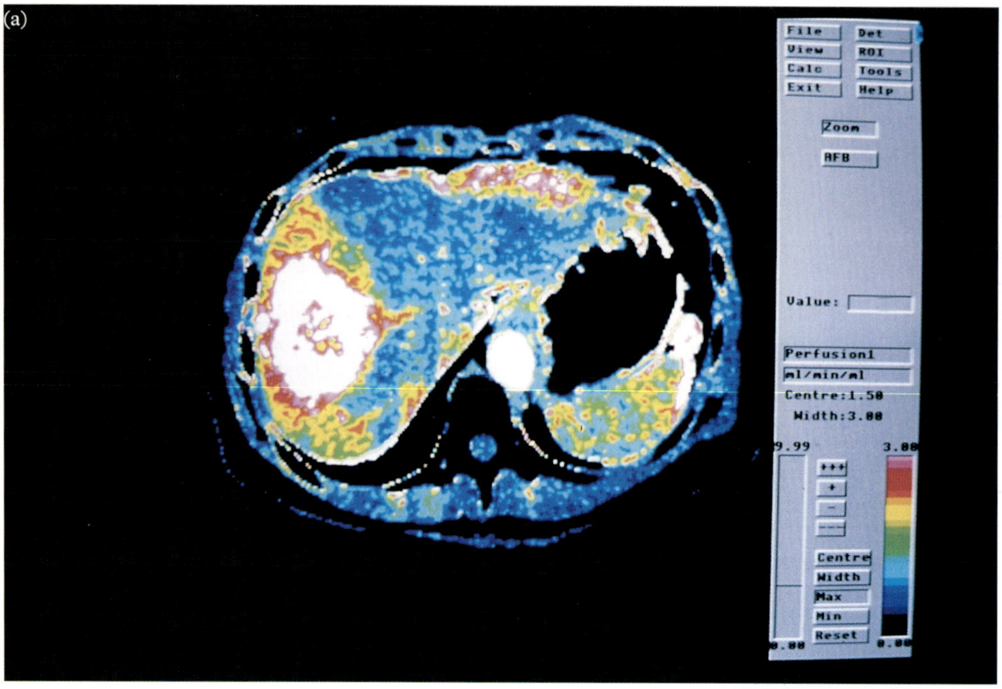

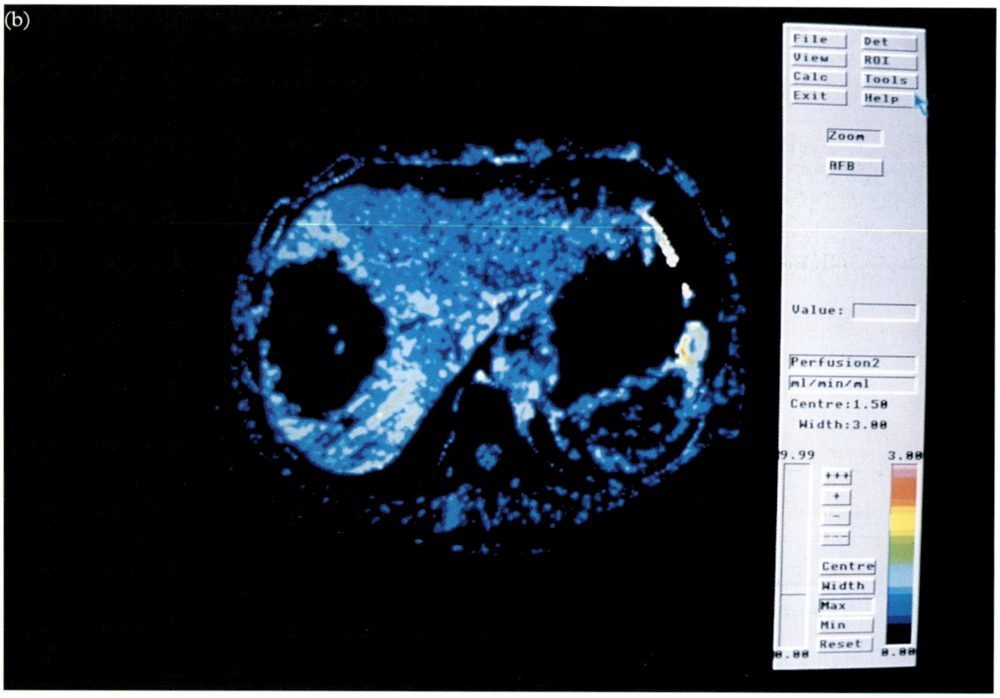

Figure 7.14
Hepatic arterial (a) and (indirect) portal (b) perfusion images of a patient with a solitary metastasis from renal carcinoma (pink: 3 ml/min/ml). Arterial perfusion is increased but portal perfusion is absent. Note that perfusion is altered adjacent to the lesion.

Figure 7.15
Tumour perfusion values before and during BW12C as assessed by perfusion CT.
= pretreatment;
= post-treatment.

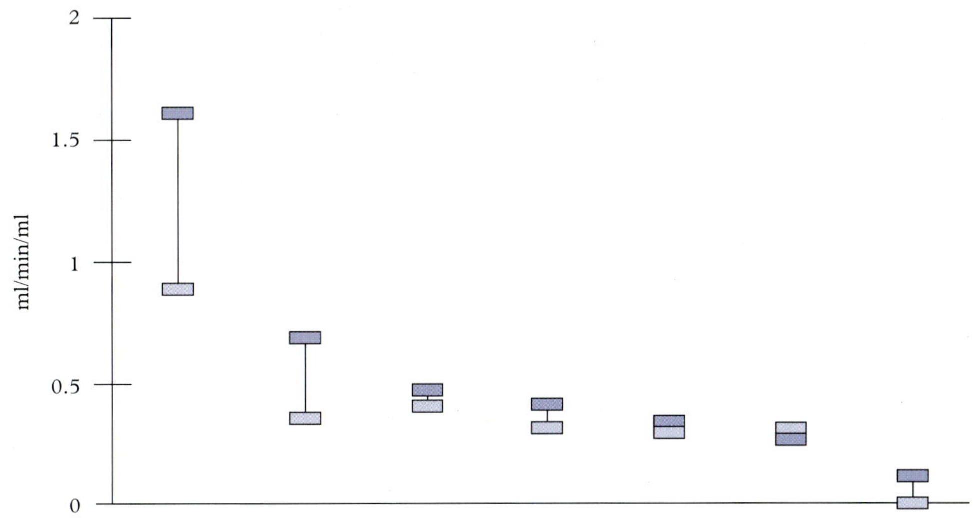

demonstrates reduced portal perfusion and this, too, is matched by the changes in the cirrhotic liver (see Figure 7.1). Detection will be consequently difficult in either phase and therefore imaging in both phases may be justified.

Oncological research has recently explored the possibility of modifying tumour perfusion pharmacologically to render the tumour more susceptible to chemotherapy or radiotherapy. Perfusion CT can be used to confirm such a change in perfusion in individual patients. Figure 7.15 demonstrates the changes in perfusion of a number of tumours before and during infusion of BW12C [29]. This agent is intended to shift the deoxyhaemoglobin saturation curve to render tumours hypoxic and therefore more susceptible to the bioreductive alkylating agent, mitomycin C. A simultaneous reduction in perfusion was found, particularly in tumours with high initial perfusion, reflecting greater delivery of the drug to the tumour. Although this fall in perfusion may increase the hypoxia, it will also reduce delivery of the chemotherapeutic agent to the tumour.

Perfusion CT can also be used to assess the severity of side effects of treatments for cancer. An example of this is given in Figure 7.16 (p. 110) which demonstrates hepatic arterial and portal perfusion images in a patient who has undergone bone-marrow transplantation. There is a marked reduction in arterial perfusion with mildly reduced portal perfusion identical to findings of rejection following liver transplantation. However, in this case, the mechanism is reversed, the native liver being rejected by the grafted marrow in a patient with graft-versus-host disease.

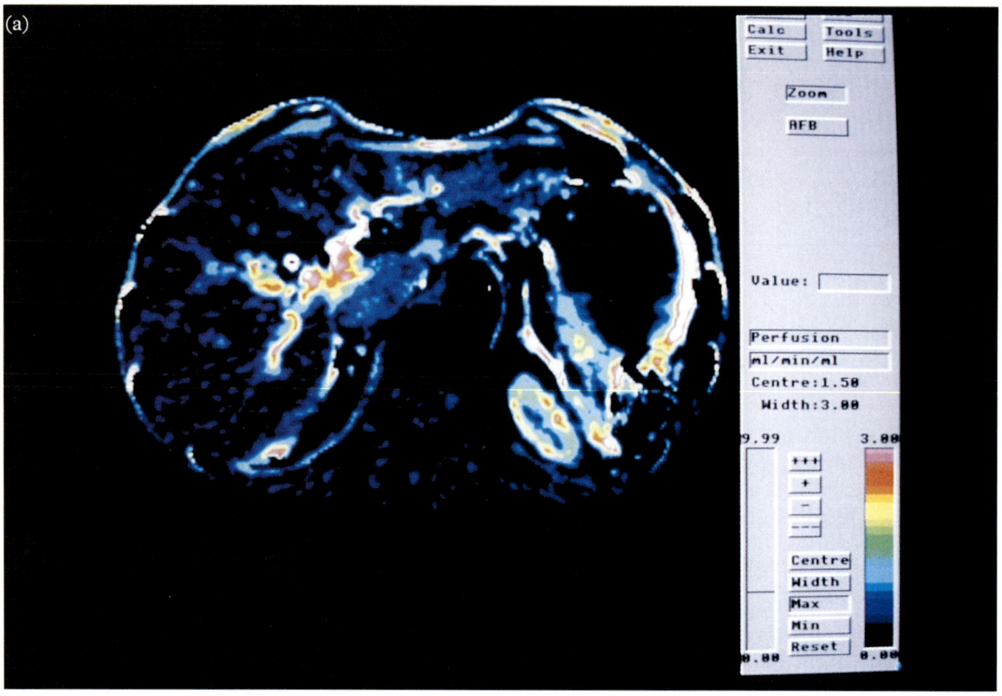

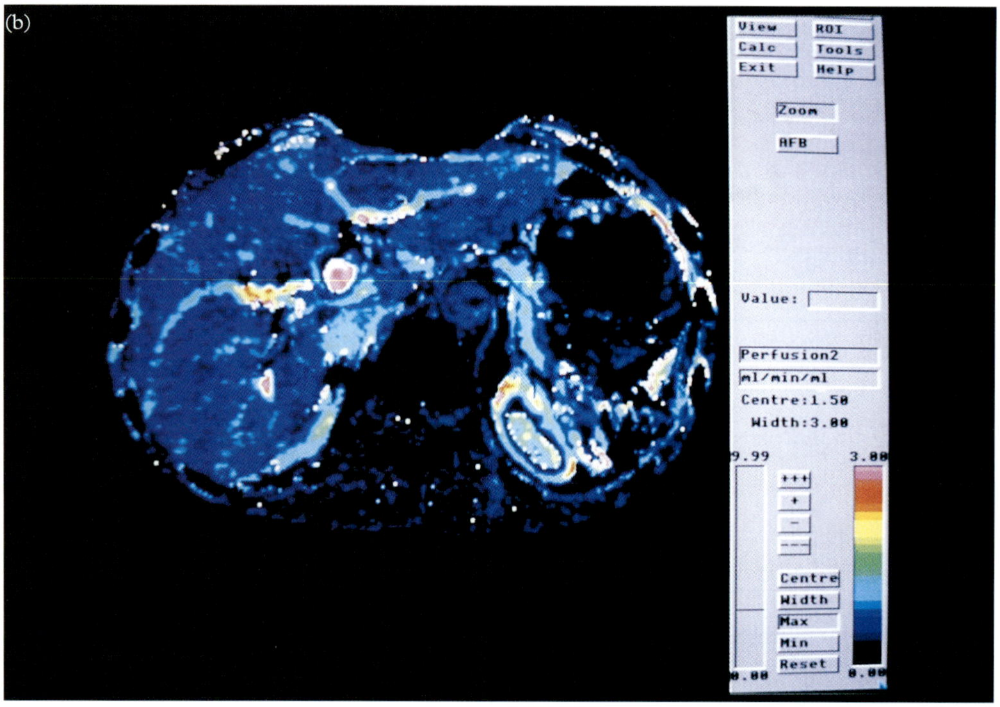

Figure 7.16
CT perfusion images of the liver in patient with graft-versus-host disease following marrow transplantation (pink: 3 ml/min/ml). Note the markedly reduced arterial perfusion (a) and low/normal portal perfusion (b) (cf. Figure 7.6).

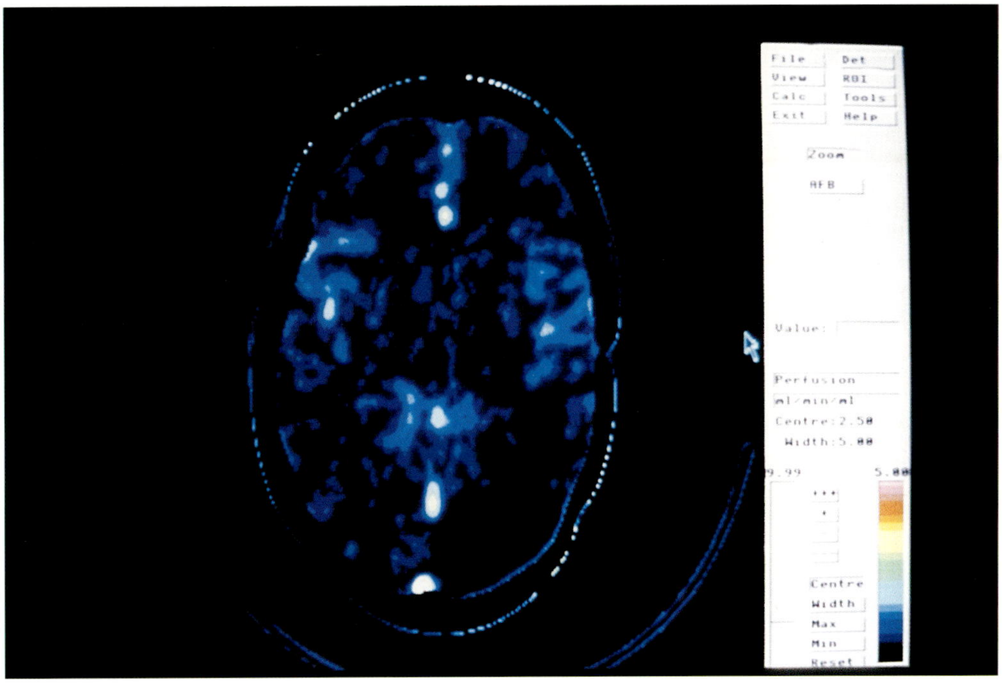

Figure 7.17
CT perfusion image (gradient method) of the brain in a patient with a left occipital infarct (pink: 5 ml/min/ml).

ACUTE AND CHRONIC BRAIN DISEASE

The first report of the use of dynamic CT to evaluate perfusion described its application to the brain [30] and it is the cerebral circulation that has been most extensively studied using such techniques. In general, the clinical applications of CT perfusion imaging of brain perfusion are no different to those demonstrated by other cerebral perfusion imaging techniques. However, the CT perfusion method may be of value in situations where the patient is already undergoing CT so that the functional information can be obtained within the same study. The additional radiation dose incurred by inclusion of a perfusion sequence is significantly lower than that associated with single-photon emission computed tomography techniques and, unlike xenon CT, perfusion CT requires no special equipment. Thus, if a contrast-enhanced CT series is to be performed, the additional perfusion information can be obtained with a low radiation burden and without compromising the overall examination. Perfusion CT may also be usefully added to CT examinations of severely ill patients, e.g. those with acute brain conditions, for whom repeated transfers to the imaging department for alternative methods of perfusion assessment could be hazardous. The technique benefits from being quantitative, allowing perfusion to be assessed in relation to ischaemic thresholds, but is constrained by its ability to study single brain slices only (even with electron beam systems or twin spiral CT machines, it is still not possible to examine the whole brain with one contrast medium injection).

There have been many studies using perfusion CT techniques to study cerebrovascular disease. Generally, these have comprised semiquantitative measures derived from gamma-fit analysis such as mean transit time (MTT), peak enhancement value and time to peak enhancement. In many reports, functional images of these parameters have been produced. Mean transit time will depend upon both the perfusion and relative blood volume of brain tissue whereas a parametric image displaying peak enhancement will be equivalent to relative perfusion (as determined by the Mullani–Gould analysis; see Chapter 4). Functional images with absolute quantification can be achieved using the gradient method [31]. Visually these are similar to relative perfusion images obtained using peak enhancement but the quantification allows comparison of perfusion with threshold values (Figure 7.17). In the acute situation, functional images may demonstrate abnormalities before any morphological change can be discerned on conventional CT images. Furthermore, the relative sizes of structural and functional abnormalities can provide useful prognostic information.

Studies applying dynamic CT to patients with cerebral vascular disease have demonstrated prolongation of MTT, reduced peak enhancement and delayed time to peak enhancement [32–36]. One group has also reported a reduction in the gradient of the upslope of cerebral time–density curves with internal carotid occlusions [37], equivalent to reduced relative perfusion as assessed by the slopes method (Chapter 4). One report attempted to distinguish patterns of cerebral vascular disease from the pattern of changes in various circulatory parameters [32]. Patients with prolonged transit and reduced peak enhancement developed massive infarction whereas prolonged transit alone was associated with partial low-density lesions on follow-up CT examinations. This interesting finding can be explained physiologically by the increased blood volume that occurs in areas of low cerebral perfusion surrounding an infarct. The increased blood volume results in prolonged transit time but the normal peak enhancement indicates preserved perfusion. In the same study, an isolated increase in the time to peak

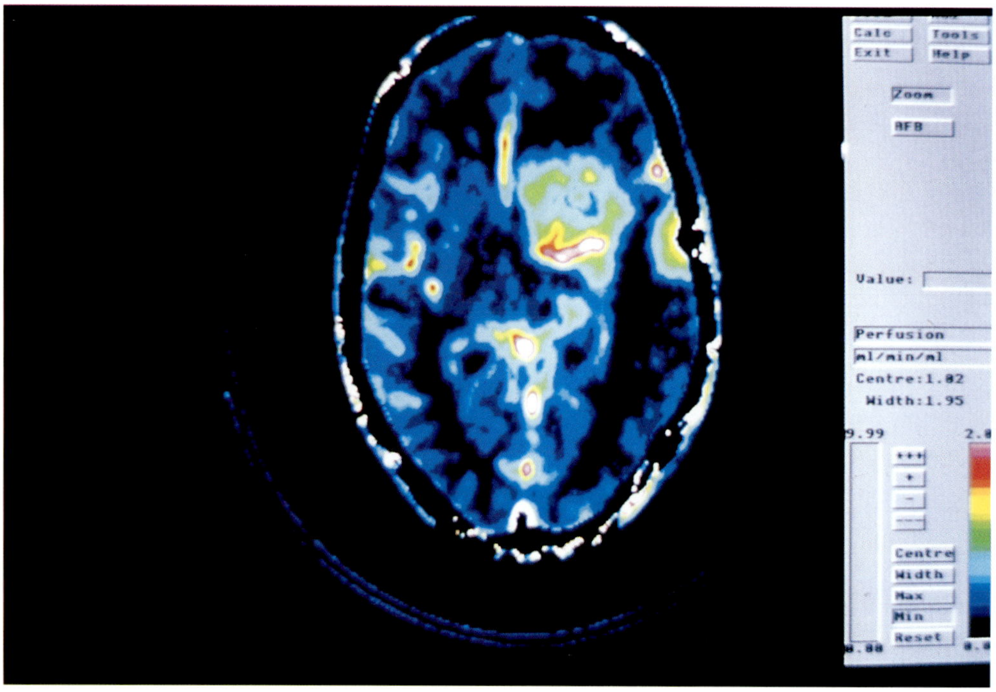

Figure 7.18
CT perfusion image of a patient with recurrent meningioma. The tumour demonstrates perfusion values higher than normal brain tissue (pink: 5 ml/min/ml).

Figure 7.19
(a) Conventional CT and (b) perfusion image of the native pancreas and pancreatic allograft in a diabetic patient (cf. Figure 6.3, page 75). The graft is a small triangular structure seen anteriorly. (arrows) There is reduced perfusion in native pancreas and graft (pink: 5 ml/min/ml).

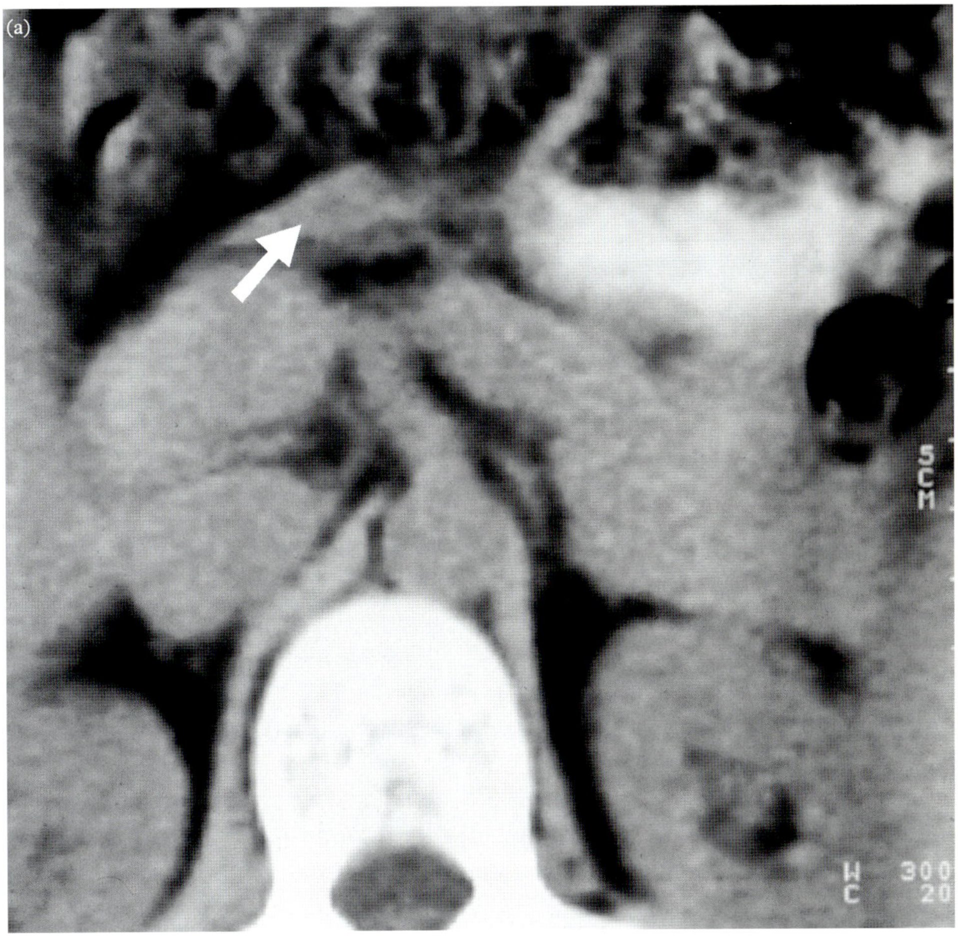

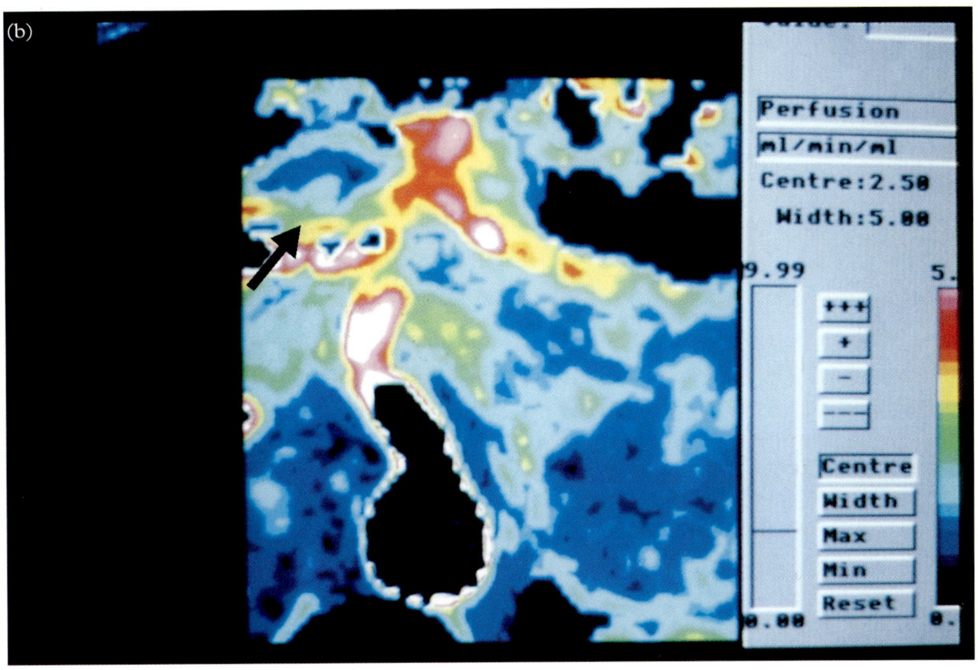

enhancement was found in patients with transient ischaemic attacks, possibly reflecting the haemodynamic effects of carotid artery stenosis. The demonstration by dynamic CT of hyperperfusion following ischaemic stroke has been reported [36] and found to be associated with a good prognosis, in keeping with the findings of PET studies. Changes in cerebral perfusion following extracranial/intracranial bypass surgery have also been reported [38].

Qualitative alterations in perfusion have been observed following head injury [39]. Hyperaemia was seen in many patients with non-fatal brain swelling, whereas most patients with subsequently fatal head injury demonstrated severe ischaemia. Other research groups have used perfusion CT to evaluate changes in perfusion associated with cranioplasty [40] and arteriovenous malformations [41]. Perfusion CT has also been used to study perfusion in meningiomas and their effects on perfusion in surrounding brain [42]. As expected, meningiomas exhibit high perfusion (Figure 7.18) whereas gliomas are relatively poorly perfused with values close to that of cerebral white matter. Perfusion has also been proposed as a marker of tumour viability in a variety of brain neoplasms [43] although permeability measurements hold greater promise in this regard (Chapter 10).

THE PANCREAS

As discussed in Chapter 6, measurement of human pancreatic perfusion has proved difficult. The difficulties in resolving small structures or reliably separating the pancreas from adjacent blood vessels can be overcome by the use of perfusion CT [44]. Figure 7.19 shows a perfusion image of the pancreas and a pancreatic graft measuring approximately 1 × 2 cm in a patient with diabetes. Compared with control subjects, perfusion values are reduced in both the native and transplanted pancreas. In the native pancreas, this can be assumed to be due to underlying diabetes that led to transplantation. In animal experiments, diabetes is associated with reduced perfusion. In this case, the reduced perfusion was considered to be due to islet-cell failure but further research is required to determine the effects of cyclosporin and rejection upon pancreatic graft perfusion.

REFERENCES

1. Sarper, R., Fajman, W.A., Rypers, E.B. *et al.* (1981) A noninvasive method for measuring portal venous/total hepatic blood flow by hepatosplenic radionuclide angiography. *Radiology*, **141**, 179–184.
2. Bolton, R.P., Mairiary, E.O., Parkin, A. *et al.* (1988) Dynamic liver scanning in cirrhosis. *Nuclear Medicine Communications*, **91**, 235–247.
3. Miles, K.A., Hayball, M.P. and Dixon, A.K. (1993) Functional images of hepatic perfusion obtained with dynamic computed tomography. *Radiology*, **188**, 405–411.
4. Blomley, M.J.K., Coulden, R., Dawson, P. *et al.* (1995) Liver perfusion studied with ultrafast CT. *Journal of Computer Assisted Tomography*, **19**(3), 424–433.
5. Shiomi, S., Kuroki, T., Ueda, T. *et al.* (1991) Measurement of hepatic blood flow by use of per-rectal portal scintigraphy with ^{133}Xe. *Nuclear Medicine Communications*, **12**, 235–242.

6. Greenway, C.V. and Lautt, W.W. (1989) Hepatic circulation. In Handbook of physiology (eds S.G. Shultz, J.D. Wood and B.B. Rauner, Bethseda, Maryland: *American Physiological Society*. Section 6, Vol. 1, Part II pp. 1519–1564.
7. Williams, R., Condon, R.E., Williams, H.S. *et al.* (1968) Splenic blood flow in cirrhosis and portal hypertension. *Clinical Science*, **34**, 441–452.
8. Gitlin, N., Grahame, G.R., Kreel, L., Williams, H.S. and Sherlock, S. (1970) Splenic blood flow and resistance in patients with cirrhosis before and after portacaval anastomoses. *Gastroenterology*, **59**, 208–213.
9. Miles, K.A., McPherson, S.J. and Hayball, M.P. (1995) Transient splenic inhomogeneity on contrast enhanced CT: mechanism and effect of liver disease. *Radiology*, **194**, 91–95.
10. Blomley, M.J.K., Coulden, R.A., Lim-Dunham, J.E. *et al.* (1997) Splenic perfusion studied with UFCT. *Academic Radiology*, **4**, 13–20.
11. Sinnatamby, R., Watson, C., Alexander, G. *et al.* (1994) Dynamic CT perfusion imaging of the transplanted liver. *British Journal of Radiology (Congress Suppl)*, **67**, 134.
12. Probst, P., Mahler, F., Roesler, H. and Fuchs, W.A. (1983) Renal artery stenosis and evaluation of the effect of endoluminal dilatation: Comparison of dynamic CT scanning and I-131-OIHA renogram. *Investigative Radiology*, **18**, 2664–2271.
13. Mukai, J. and Sabel, P. (1986) Application of dynamic computed tomography to physiologic imaging of renal artery stenosis before and after angioplasty. *American Journal of Physiological Imaging*, **1**, 33–43.
14. Heinz, E.R., Dubois, P.J., Drayer, B.P. and Hall, R. (1980) A preliminary investigation of dynamic computed tomography in renovascular hypertension. *Journal of Computer Assisted Tomography*, **4**, 63–66.
15. Miles, K.A. (1991) Measurement of tissue perfusion by dynamic computed tomography. *British Journal of Radiology* **64**, 409–412.
16. Gruenewald, S.M., Nimmon, C.C., Nawaz, M.K. and Britton, K.E. (1981) A non-invasive γ-camera technique for the measurement of intrarenal flow distribution in man. *Clinical Science*, **61**, 385–389.
17. Blomley, M.J.K., Albrecht, T., Jåger, H.R. *et al.* (1995) Functional perfusion imaging: a potentially useful adjunct to spiral CT. *British Journal of Radiology, (Rontgen Centenary Congress)*, 107.
18. Ishikawa, I., Masuzaki, S., Saito, T. *et al.* (1985) Dynamic computed tomography in acute renal failure: analysis of time–density curve. *Journal of Computer Assisted Tomography*, **9**, 1097–1102.
19. Jaschke, W.R., Sievers, R., Lipton, M.J. and Cogan, M.G. (1989) Cine-computed tomographic assessment of regional renal blood flow. *Acta Radiologica*, **31**, 77–81.
20. Blomley, M.J.K., Kormano, M., Coulden, R. *et al.* (1994) Renal perfusion quantified with contrast enhanced CT. *Investigative Radiology*, **29**(2), S232–233.
21. Miles, K.A., London, N.J.M., Lavelle, J.M. *et al.* (1991) CT staging of renal carcinoma: a prospective study of three dynamic computed tomography techniques. *European Journal of Radiology*, **13**, 37–42.
22. Fuld, I.L., Matalon, T.A., Vogelzang, R.L. *et al.* (1984) Dynamic CT in the evaluation of physiologic status of renal transplants. *American Journal of Roentgenology*, **142**, 1157–1160.
23. Jansen, V.O., Gmelin, E., Burmester, E. *et al.* (1989) Analyse von dynamischen CT-kurven bei nierentransplantaten mit abstossungsreaktion und cyclosporin-A-intoxikation. *ROFO*, **151**, 473–476.
24. Miles, K.A., Hayball, M.P. and Dixon, A.K. (1994) Functional imaging of changes in human intrarenal perfusion using quantitative dynamic computed tomography. *Investigative Radiology*, **29**, 911–914.
25. Hattori, H., Miyoski, T., Okada, J. *et al.* (1994) Tumor blood flow measured using dynamic computed tomography. *Investigative Radiology*, **29**, 873–876.

26. Hosoki, T. (1983) Dynamic CT of pancreatic tumours. *American Journal of Roentgenology*, **140**, 959–965.
27. Groell, R., Kugler, C., Aschauer, M. *et al.* (1995) Quantitative perfusion parameters of focal nodular hyperplasia and normal liver parenchyma as determined by electron beam tomography. *British Journal of Radiology*, **68**, 1185–1193.
28. Leen, E., Wilson, W.J., Wotherspoon, H. *et al.* (1995) Detection of colorectal liver metastases: comparison of laparotomy, CT, US and Doppler perfusion index and evaluation of postoperative follow-up results. *Radiology*, **195**, 113–116.
29. Falk, S.J., Ramsay, J.R., Ward, R. *et al.* (1994) BW12C perturbs normal and tumour tissue oxygenation and blood flow in man. *Radiotherapy and Oncology*, **32**, 210–217.
30. Axel, L. (1980) Cerebral blood flow determination by rapid-sequence computed tomography; theoretical analysis. *Radiology*, **137**, 679–686.
31. Sinnatamby, R., Miles, K.A., Hayball, M.P. and Dixon, A.K. (1994) CT perfusion imaging of the brain: iodine or xenon? *British Journal of Radiology*, (*Congress Suppl*), **67**, 135.
32. Nagata, K. and Asano, T. (1990) Functional image of dynamic computed tomography for the evaluation of cerebral hemodynamics. *Stroke*, **21**, 882–899.
33. Nakayasu, H., Sue, S., Hikasa, C. and Takahashi, K. (1991) Dynamic computed tomography and functional imaging in cerebral arterial occlusive disease: analysis in the chronic phase. *Acta Neurologica Scandinavica*, **84**, 243–249.
34. Shih, T.T.F. and Huang, K-M. (1988) Acute stroke: detection of changes in cerebral perfusion with dynamic CT scanning. *Radiology*, **169**, 469–474.
35. Davis, S.M., Tress, B.M., Hopper, J.L., Kaye, A.H. and Rossiter, S.C. (1987) Dynamic CT brain scanning in the haemodynamic evaluation of cerebral arterial occlusive disease. *Neuroradiology*, **29**, 259–265.
36. Traupe, H., Heiss, W.D., Hoeffken, W. and Zuich, K.J. (1979) Hyperperfusion and enhancement in dynamic computed tomography of ischemic stroke patients. *Journal of Computer Assisted Tomography*, **3**, 627–632.
37. Heinz, E.R., Dubois, P., Osborne, D., Drayer, B. and Barrett, W. (1979) Dynamic computed tomography study of the brain. *Journal of Computer Assisted Tomography*, **3**, 641–649.
38. Takahashi, N., Kikuchi, H. and Karasawa, J. (1983) Dynamic CT in patients with superficial temporal-middle cerebral artery anastomosis. *American Journal of Neuroradiology*, **4**, 454–457.
39. Yoshino, E., Yamaki, T., Higuchi, T., Horikawa, Y. and Hirakawa, K. (1985) Acute brain edema in fatal head injury: analysis by dynamic CT scanning. *Journal of Neurosurgery*, **63**, 830–839.
40. Suzuki, N., Suzuki, S. and Iwabuchi, T. (1993) Neurological improvement after cranioplasty. Analysis by dynamic CT scan. *Acta Neurochir (Wien)*, **122**, 49–53.
41. Handa, J., Matsuda, M., Nakasu, Y., Nakasu, S. and Morioka, Y. (1983) Dynamic computed tomography and functional imaging in cerebral vascular anomalies. *Surgical Neurology*, **19**, 497–507.
42. Jinkins, J.R. and Sener, R.N. (1991) The characteristics of cerebral meningiomas and surrounding tissues on dynamic CT. *Neuroradiology*, **33**, 499–506.
43. Nakagomi, T. and Takakura, K. (1984) Dynamic computed tomography of brain tumor (in Japanese) *No To Shinkei*, **36**, 1031–1040.
44. Miles, K.A., Hayball, M.P. and Dixon, A.K. (1995) Measurement of human pancreatic perfusion using dynamic computed tomography with perfusion imaging. *British Journal of Radiology*, **68**, 471–475.

Chapter 8

MEASUREMENT OF RENAL FUNCTION BY CT

P. Dawson

The kidneys play a crucial role in the excretion of waste products but have an equally important role in the control of the milieu in which all cells of the body are located. The kidneys modulate the volume, osmolality and electrolyte concentrations in this milieu. Hence the importance of the assessment of renal function of both native and transplant kidneys. There are a number of reasons why the measurement of renal function during an imaging investigation might be clinically useful, particularly in oncology where many patients require extensive imaging, including computed tomography (CT), for staging and follow-up during and after treatment. Such patients may be undergoing concomitant treatment with nephrotoxic drugs, necessitating the monitoring of renal function; the doses of some cytotoxic drugs may need consequent modification in the light of any renal functional impairment; obstructive uropathy is not uncommon in malignant disease of the abdomen and pelvis and assessment of its functional significance is important; and renal-function impairment is often poorly assessed by measurements of urea and creatinine. More generally, in routine practice, many patients with actual or potential renal disease undergo CT or need an X-ray contrast injection for other reasons. If adjunct functional information could be obtained at the same attendance, this would be desirable.

The use of X-ray contrast agents as tracers would seem a promising approach as the kidney is a 'target' organ for these agents in that the kidney is effectively the sole site of their elimination from the body by passive glomerular filtration, all other processes being of minimal importance even in the face of significant renal impairment [1].

The poor track record of the intravenous urogram [IVU] (Figure 8.1) as a reliable indicator of renal function does not provide a promising pointer to the successful use of imaging techniques but a better understanding of contrast agent pharmacokinetics, dynamic imaging and more sophisticated mathematical analyses have now changed the situation dramatically.

We have already seen in Chapter 3 how measurements of plasma contrast/iodine concentration measurements made at later times (approximately 1.5 hours) may be used to obtain an estimate of glomerular filtration rate (GFR)/unit volume extracellular fluid (ECF) from the slope of a semi-log plot [1,2–5]. This is a fundamental measurement of GFR of considerable

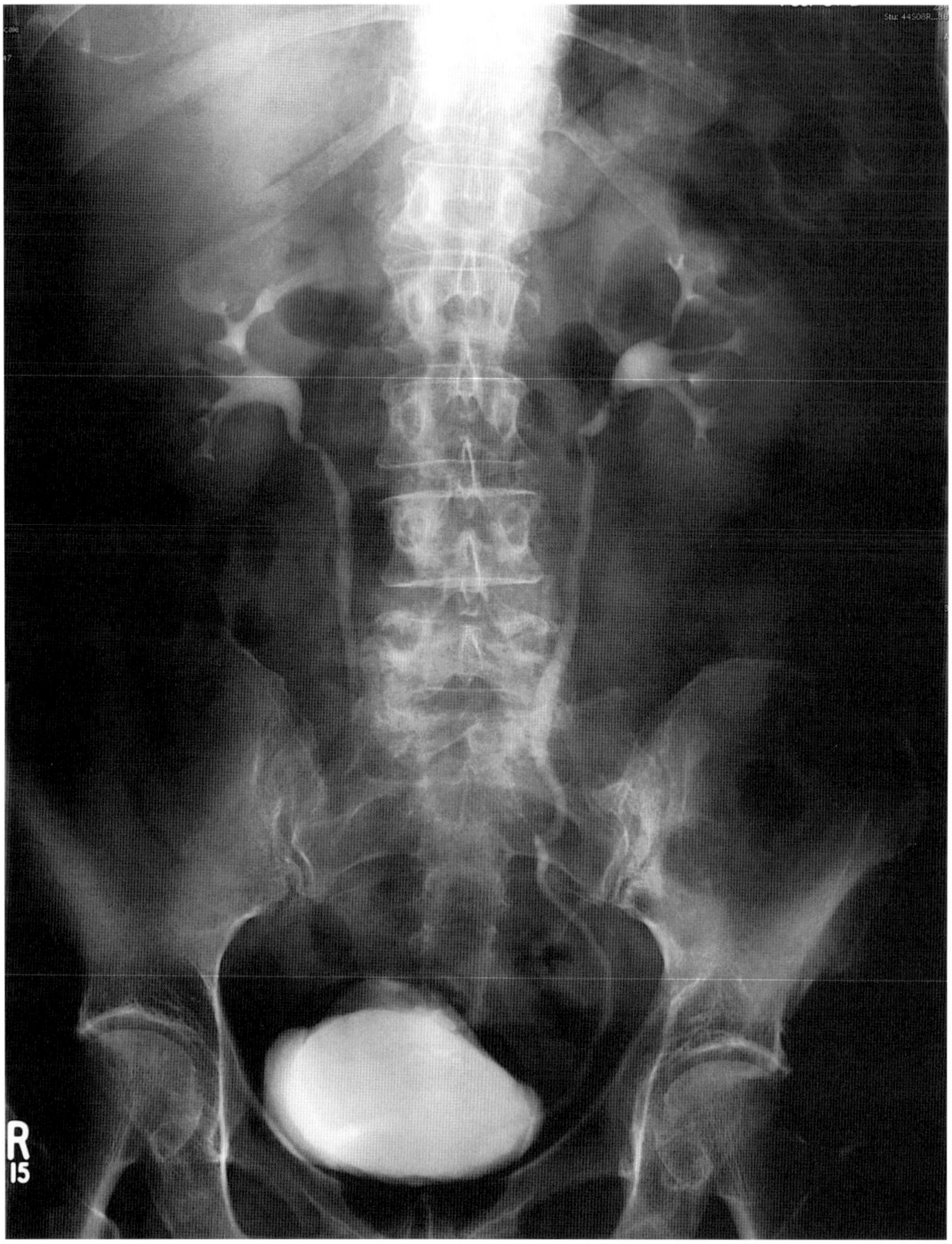

Figure 8.1
A traditional IVU is of very limited value in assessing renal function, yet real data on this are hidden in such images.

physiological interest and importance, but the disadvantages of the method are several-fold: there is delay and inconvenience to the patient; blood samples must be taken, spun down and plasma separated. However, the process is simplified by the availability of dedicated X-ray fluorescence equipment for the measurements [1]. The method has even been used with gadolinium chelates as the tracer substance indicating that assessment of renal function during magnetic resonance imaging (MRI) examinations is possible [2].

It has been further shown that if the total dose of contrast administered is large then background-subtracted CT N°s taken from a large region of interest (ROI)

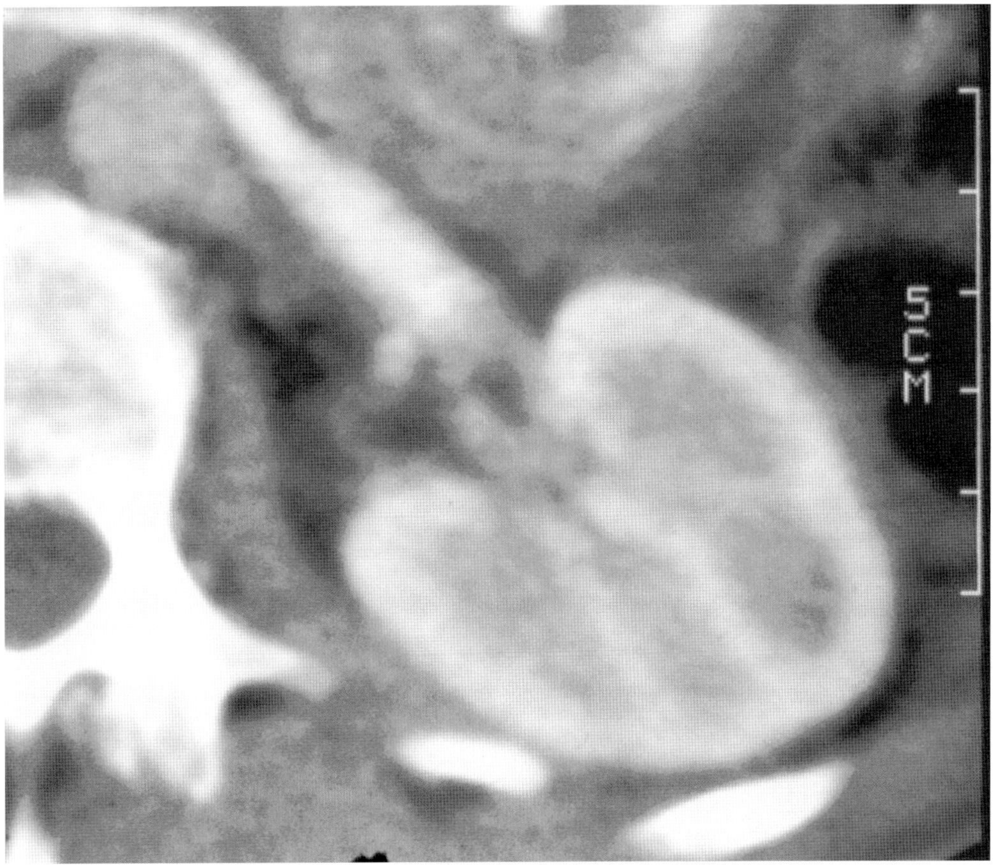

Figure 8.2
A single CT image of a kidney from a sequence taken following intravenous bolus contrast injection. A cortical nephrogram is well developed. A series of such images/datasets contain a good deal of usually neglected physiological and microanatomical information.

in the aorta may be used in the semi-log plot [2]. However, the signal-to-noise ratio is not high in this method.

In this chapter, we examine an approach to the assessment of renal function using dynamic CT image data from the kidney following a peripheral venous bolus injection of a modest amount (25 ml) of contrast agent in a manner akin to that used for the perfusion measurements described in Chapters 5 to 7. Indeed, much the same dataset may be used for both measurements.

Figure 8.2 shows a single image of the kidney from a dynamic sequence taken following peripheral venous contrast injection. An excellent cortical nephrogram is seen [6]. As discussed in Chapter 3, even at an early stage of its development a nephrogram like this is the net result of contrast agent in the blood (plasma) pool and contrast agent in tubules following first-pass filtration [6,7]. The interstitial component is anatomically small and is effectively part of the blood-pool volume because of the high permeability of renal capillaries [8].

The challenge is to unravel these two components from the curves. The time evolution of the relative contributions of the two compartments reflects filtration from the one to the other, indicating that, in principle, data on GFR is hidden in the curves. The concentration of contrast (CT N°) in a renal artery or adjacent aorta clearly gives information about the blood-pool concentration [6,7,9–11] and an approach to the problem using this fact is now described.

THEORETICAL BACKGROUND

If we assume glomerular filtration to be a linear process, then:

$$-\frac{\mathrm{d}Q(t)}{\mathrm{d}t} = \alpha b(t) \tag{1}$$

where $Q(t)$ is the contrast mass at time, t, in the circulation, $b(t)$ its blood concentration at that time and α the GFR (Figure 8.3).

Therefore, the mass transferred out of the blood into tubules by time, t, will be:

$$Q(t) = \alpha \int_0^t b(t)\mathrm{d}t \tag{2}$$

If we divide by V, the volume of the ROI under consideration, we obtain:

$$\frac{Q(t)}{V} = \frac{\alpha}{V}\int_0^t b(t)\mathrm{d}t \tag{3}$$

This represents the contribution at any time, t, to the total concentration in the ROI of filtered contrast.

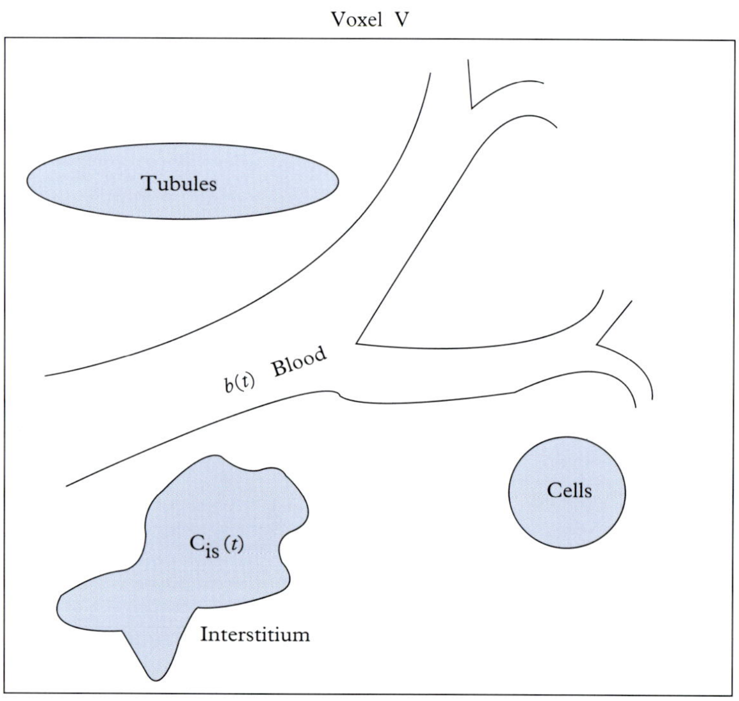

Figure 8.3
The anatomical compartments of the kidney. The interstitium is small and, effectively, part of the blood pool because of the high vascular permeability in the kidney.

The contribution of the contrast remaining at time t in blood is

$$\phi_b b(t)$$

where ϕ_b is the proportion of the volume, V, of the ROI which is blood. The total effective concentration, $c(t)$, in the kidney ROI is therefore

$$c(t) = \frac{\alpha}{V}\int_0^t b(t)\mathrm{d}t + \phi_b b(t) \tag{4}$$

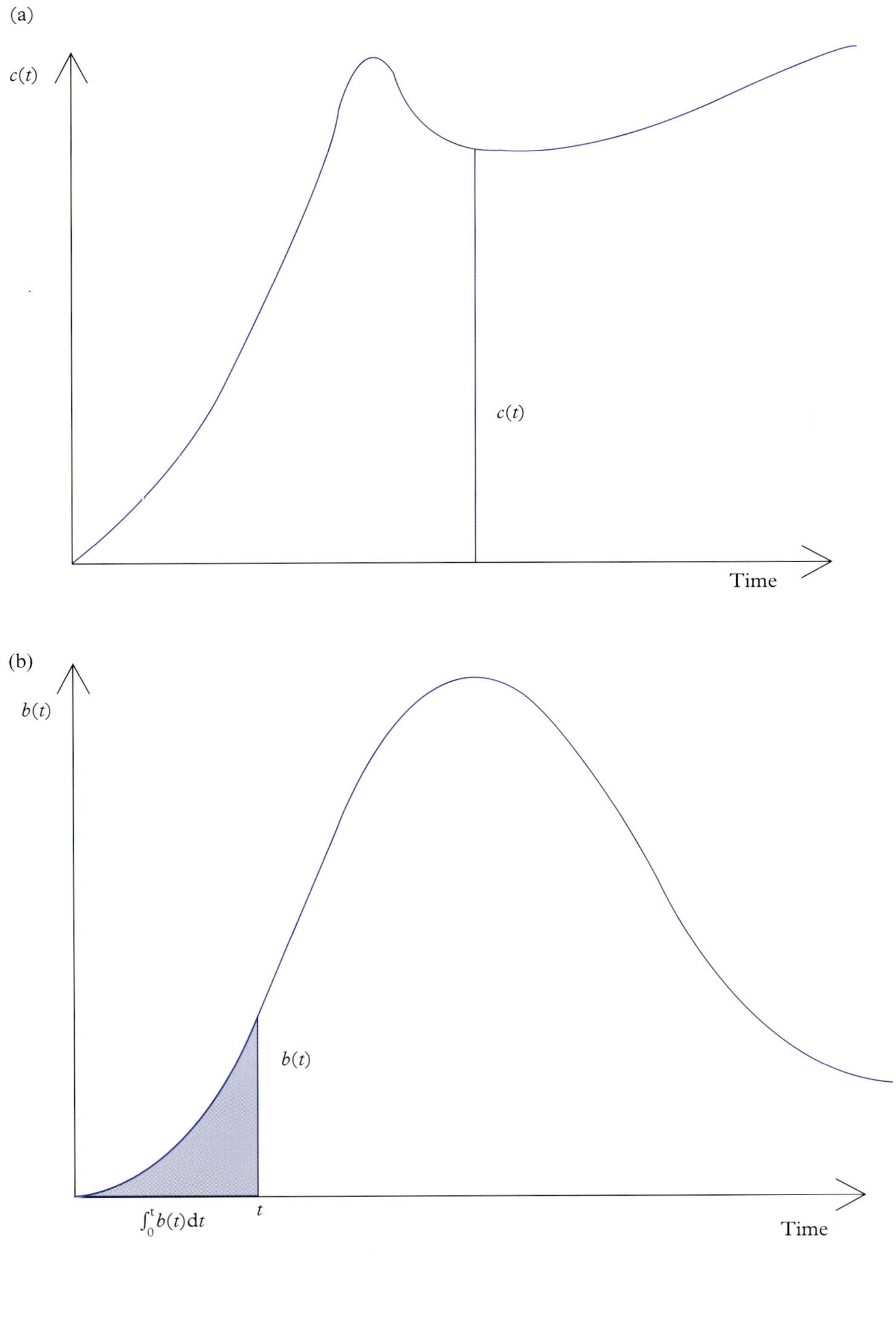

Figure 8.4
(a) The renal ROI versus time curve. $c(t)$ may be simply read off for any t. (b) The arterial input curve. $b(t)$ may be simply read off. $\int_0^t b(t)\mathrm{d}t$ is the area shaded which may be calculated by the trapezium rule.

If we divide by $b(t)$:

$$\frac{c(t)}{b(t)} = \frac{\frac{\alpha}{V}\int_0^t b(t)\mathrm{d}t}{b(t)} + \phi_b \tag{5}$$

This mathematical manoeuvre, previously discussed in Chapter 4, was developed by Patlak and colleagues for positron emission tomography (PET) studies of the brain [7,12] and has been adapted for nuclear medicine studies of the kidney in some centres. As we have noted, because of their linearity, background-subtracted CT N°s may be substituted for concentrations in these equations. This is the key to the application of the method to dynamic CT. $c(t)$ becomes the CT N° of the usual tissue ROI, $b(t)$ the CT N° in a nearby artery, renal artery or aorta. $\int_0^t b(t)\mathrm{d}t$ is the area under the arterial curve up to time t (Figure 8.4a,b). The units of $\int_0^t b(t)\mathrm{d}t$ will be CT N° $\times$ time.

Thus

$$\frac{\int_0^t b(t)\mathrm{d}t}{b(t)}$$

will have units of time. The entity is sometimes called 'Patlak time' [7,12].

$c(t)/b(t)$ plotted against $\int_0^t b(t)\mathrm{d}t/b(t)$ will be linear with gradient α/V and intercept on the ordinate of ϕ_b. This is illustrated diagramatically in Figure 8.5.

Since $c(t)/b(t)$ is unitless, the gradient, α/V, will be in units of inverse time. Figure 8.4(a,b) indicates diagramatically how $b(t)$, $c(t)$ and $\int_0^t b(t)\mathrm{d}t$ may be obtained from the dynamic CT data.

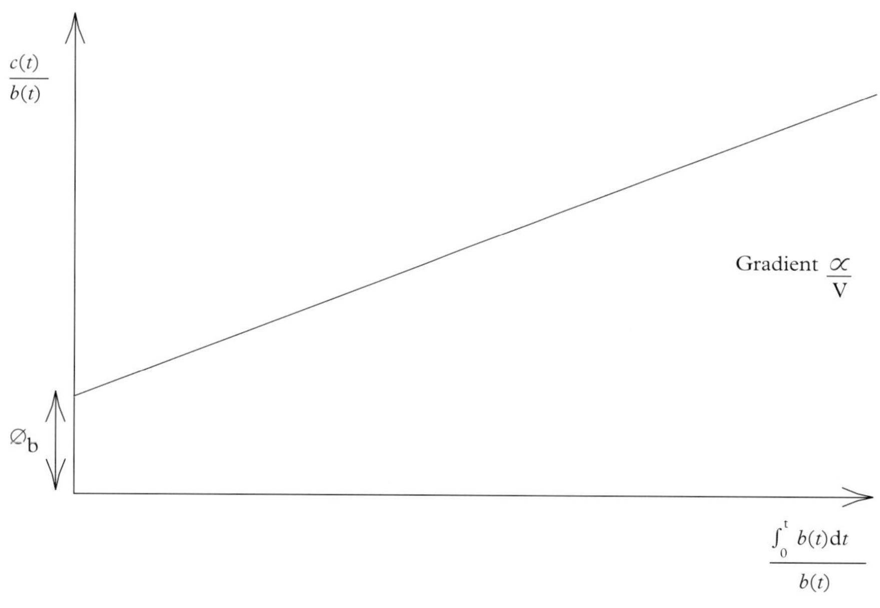

Figure 8.5
A diagrammatic Patlak plot.

TECHNIQUE

Non-ionic contrast agent (25 ml) is administered by rapid bolus injection at 5 ml/s using a pump connected to a cannula in an antecubital vein. The non-ionic agent is chosen so as to minimize haemodynamic and other changes as discussed in Chapter 3 (page 43).

A single-axial 10 mm slice is taken through the middle of the kidney. Half-way through the injection the sequence of images through the fixed section is started and continued at 5 s intervals for approximately 1 min. The patient is allowed to breathe gently throughout this period. Arterial contrast density–time curves and renogram contrast density–time curves are then generated from ROIs in the abdominal aorta and in the kidney. The kidney ROIs may be the whole kidney, the cortex or any volume down to pixel level [7]. The precontrast images are subtracted from each of the dynamic images to yield background-subtracted CT N°–time curves for aortic and renal ROIs and the Patlak plots then performed according to the prescription of Equation(6).

Typical curves for aorta and whole kidney are shown in Figure 8.6 and, for comparison, analogous curves from a nuclear medicine study with Tc DTPA are shown in Figure 8.7 (a,b). The similarities are unsurprising but encouraging.

A typical Patlak plot of real data is shown in Figure 8.8. The correlation coefficient of the regression line of the data in this case is 0.97, a figure typical in these studies. Also typical of such studies is an intercept on the ordinate of about 0.3, representing the proportionate vascular volume which will be discussed further below.

The gradient of the curve is a measure of GFR per unit volume of kidney and in Figure 8.8 a typical value of 0.45 is found. Because of the novel nature of the measurement, such figures are not readily comparable with the usual data on GFR but suffice it to say, for the moment, that it is a fundamental measurement worthy of close attention.

Quality of the data

Given that the patients are allowed to breathe during the examination and that only 25 ml of contrast is given, the quality of the data and fit obtainable is outstanding.

Proportionate vascular volume

Values obtained in a variety of patients range from 0.27 to 0.31. Such values appear entirely plausible for a vascular organ such as the kidney. However, a caveat needs to be entered regarding any assumption of the validity for the kidney of a two-compartment model — there is a small interstitium in the kidney which communicates so freely with the blood pool through highly permeable arterioles as to be part of it. The figure obtained from the Patlak-plot intercept is therefore a slight overestimate of blood volume). Strictly speaking, contrast is present in three compartments in the kidney: vascular, interstitial and tubular. Depending on the rate at which contrast equilibrates between vascular and interstitial compartments, the slope of the Patlak plot may include a component of clearance into the interstitial space in addition to glomerular filtration. Tc DTPA

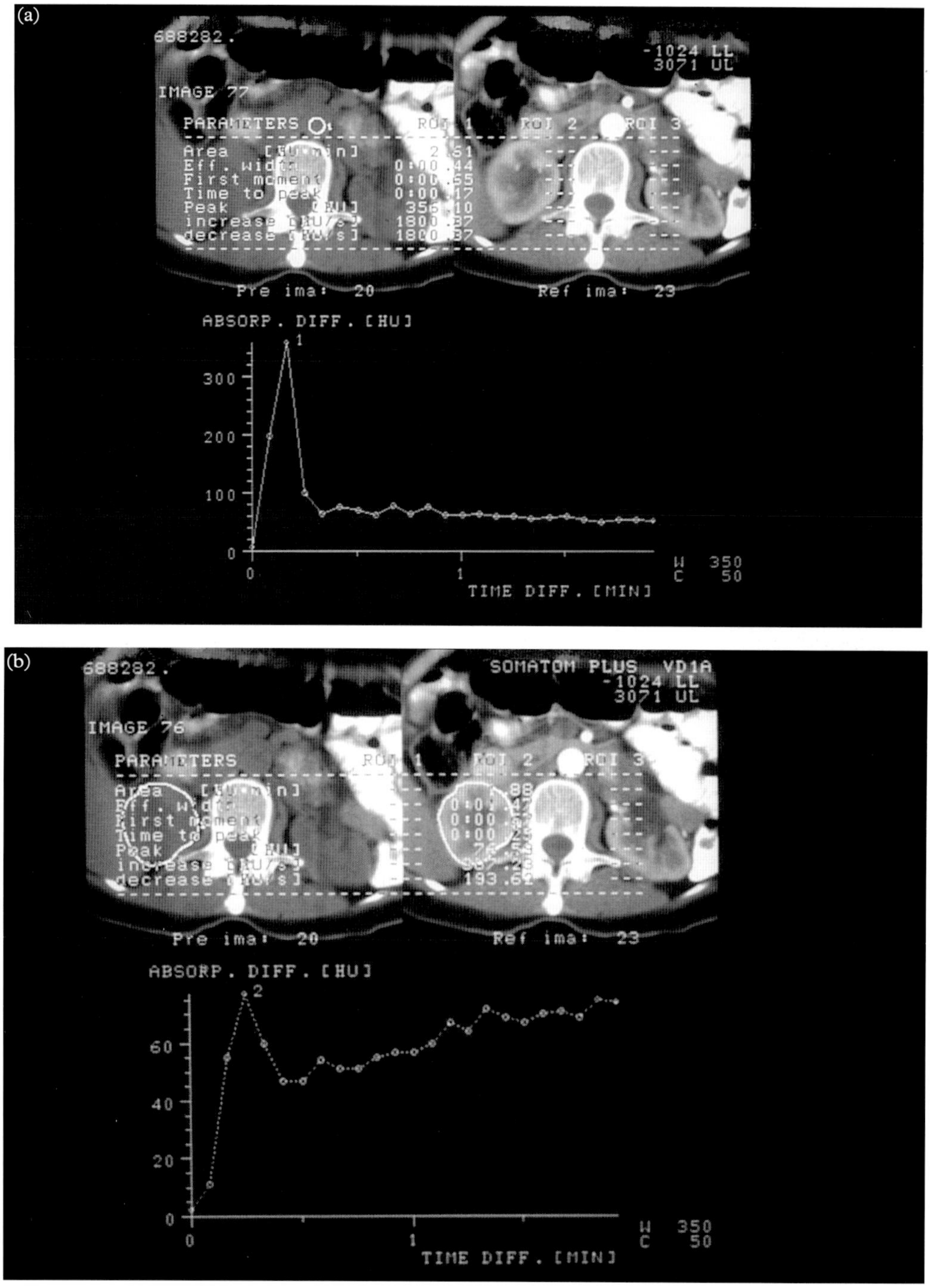

Figure 8.6
Typical aortic (a) and renal (b) ROI CT N° versus time curves. Data points acquired at 5 s intervals.

equilibrates relatively slowly between intravascular and extravascular spaces of muscle and skin [13,14]. Therefore, for about 2 min after intravenous injection, outflow of DTPA into the extravascular space of muscle and skin greatly exceeds backflow, and so the contribution made by clearance of Tc DTPA, from vascular space to interstitial fluid of background tissue, is clearly evident in the slope of the Patlak plot of the unsubtracted DTPA renogram. The peritubular capillaries of the kidney, however, have a much higher permeability to small hydrophilic

Figure 8.7
(a), (b) Tc DTPA renogram exhibiting the same form as the CT N° curve. This is to be expected since the pharmacokinetics are the same and in each case the 'signal' parameter is proportional to concentration.

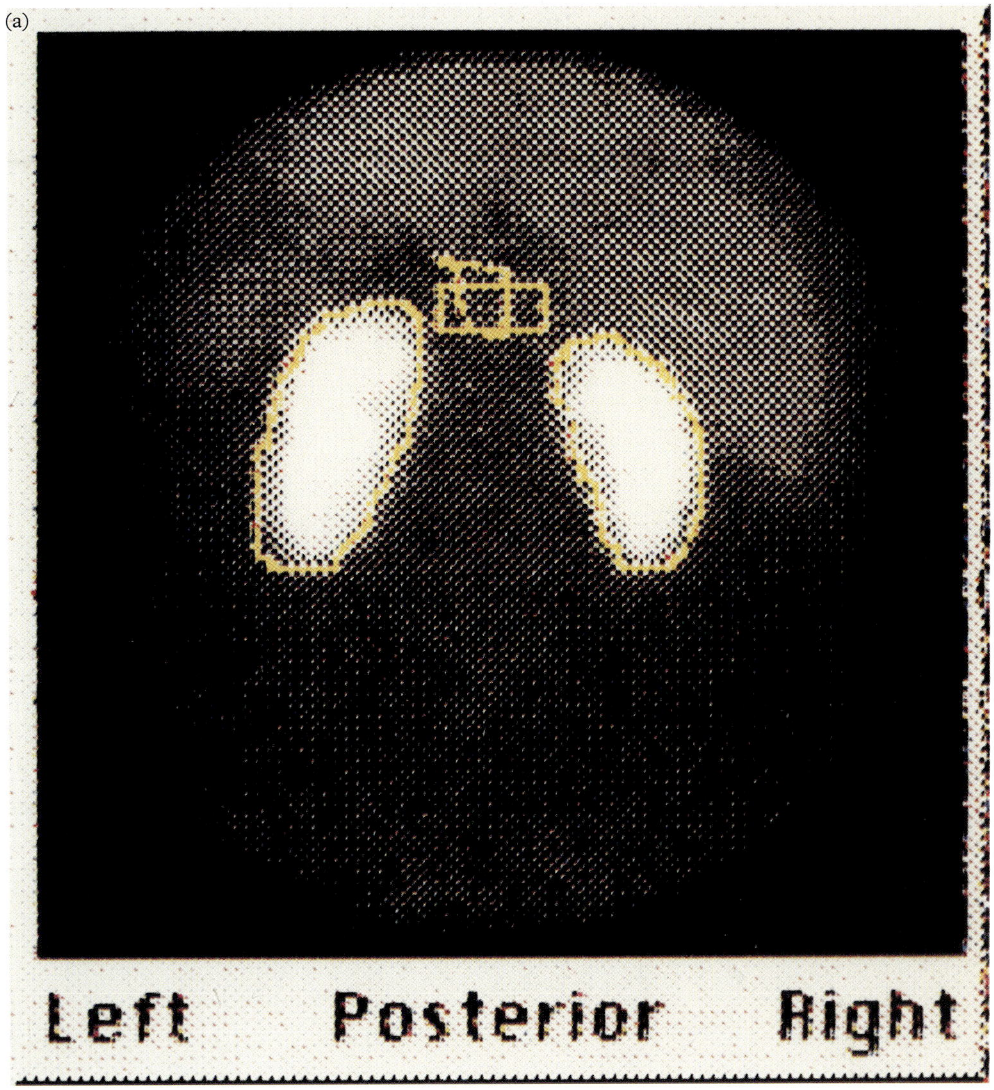

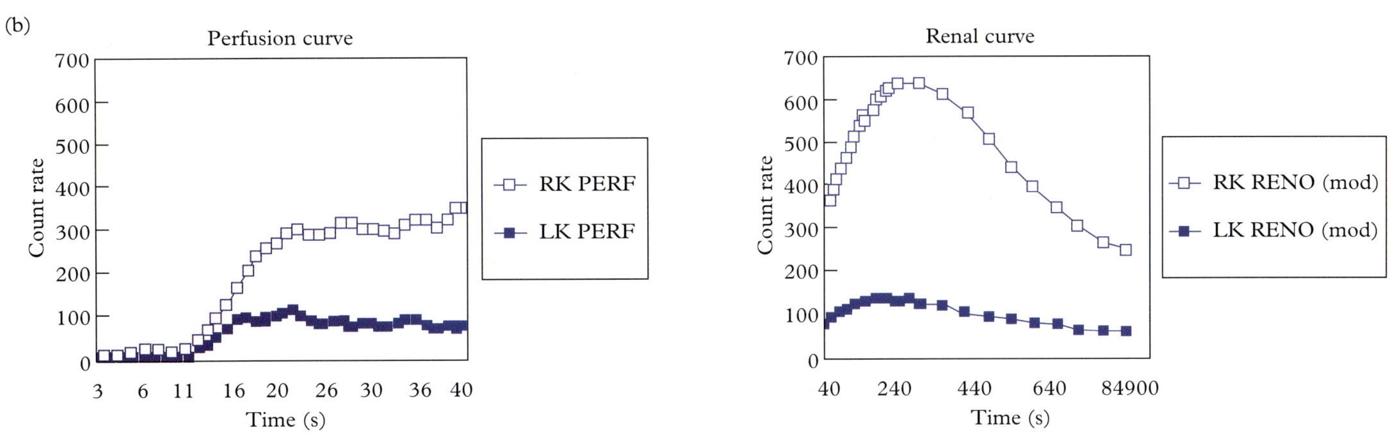

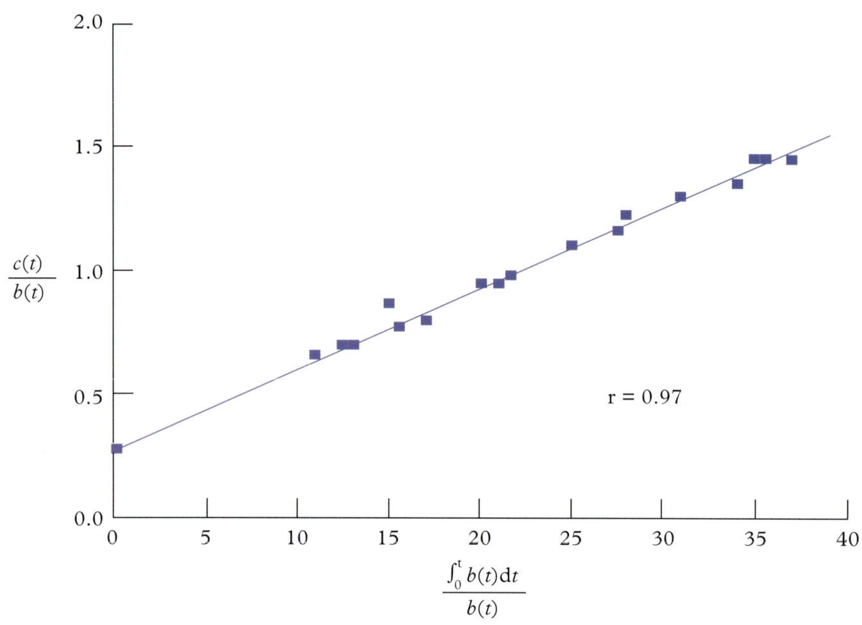

Figure 8.8
A Patlak plot of the data of Figure 8.6. The correlation coefficient of the regression is 0.97, an indication of the quality of data obtainable. The intercept of ~ 0.3 on the ordinate indicates the proportionate vascular volume of the kidney.

solutes [8] which, along with the relatively much smaller interstitial volume in the kidney would promote a much more rapid equilibration rate as compared with skin and muscles. It is likely, therefore, that the Patlak plot slope represents GFR while the intercept on the ordinate includes renal interstitial volume, which may be expected therefore to be a slight overestimate. Interestingly, however, the range 0.27 to 0.31 is entirely compatible with the value of 28% obtained by Hillman *et al.* [15] in experiments using an experimental blood-pool agent.

Such an interpretation is supported by the linearity of Patlak plots carried out on data up to 2 or 3 min following contrast injection at which time contrast begins to enter the outflow tract and leave the kidney.

Patlak plot slope and GFR

The value obtained by this method for the Patlak slope of Figure 8.8 is 0.45 ml/min/ml. Normal single-kidney inulin blood clearance is approximately 100 ml per minute which in a kidney with a volume of 150 ml would yield a GFR value per unit volume of approximately 0.67 ml/min/ml. This indicates that this particular patient had a modestly reduced level of renal function. However, it should be noted that no normal range has yet been established for this novel parameter.

Mean transit time

Interestingly, the data from such studies can be used to estimate a value for the mean transit time (MTT) through the kidney which is a parameter of considerable interest, as discussed in Chapter 4, in assessing the accuracy of the several algorithms for calculation of perfusion.

Renal blood flow to each kidney is some 10% of cardiac output, i.e. some 0.5 *l*/min = 0.5/60 *l*/s. The volume of blood in the kidneys is proportionate to vascular volume × renal volume. This is approximately 0.3×150 ml = 50 ml = 0.05 *l*.

Applying the central volume theorem to these data [4,16], we may say the MTT for the kidney is

$$\text{MTT} = \frac{\text{Renal blood volume}}{\text{Blood flow}}$$

$$= \frac{0.05}{(0.5/60)} = 6\,\text{s}$$

This is an intriguing and reassuring result. As discussed in Chapter 4, it is essential that in the peak and peak gradient methods, the time to reach peak and peak gradient, respectively, must not exceed the minimum transit time in the organ. Clearly, since the peak gradient is reached before the peak, the method utilizing this is less critically dependent on the transit time assumption. A figure of 6 s for the MTT suggests that the gradient method may be reliably applied to renal-perfusion measurements but that the peak method may not be. This is reflected in the results from the two methods which indicate that the gradient approach produces data close to 'gold-standard' invasive methods but that the peak method underestimates perfusion significantly [9].

THE NEPHROGRAM

The nature of the nephrogram (Figures 8.2 and 8.9) is a very old conundrum but is of more than passing academic significance since it may be abnormal in a number of characteristic ways in renal disease [17]. Thus, in chronic glomerular disease there is frequently a faint but persistent nephrogram. In acute obstruction there is often an increasingly dense nephrogram; in acute tubular necrosis an immediate dense and persistent nephrogram is described. A persistent nephrogram seen at CT 24 h after an arteriogram in a patient with contrast-agent associated acute-on-chronic renal failure is illustrated in Figure 8.10. An understanding of the physiology and pathophysiology of contrast handling and distribution in the kidney in health and disease, as reflected by the nephrogram, will therefore be of clinical as well as academic importance.

The technique described and the data it generates allow us to answer the basic question concerning the nature of the normal nephrogram readily. Once the intercept, ϕ_b, is determined it may be used as a scaling factor on the arterial curve. Since CT N°s are linear, we may subtract this scaled arterial curve from the organ curve, thereby obtaining a filtrate curve (Figure 8.11). We can then determine by simple inspection of these curves the relative contributions at any moment of blood pool and filtrate. It may be seen from Figure 8.11, which is such a plot for a normal kidney, that the blood-pool contribution continues to be significant up to 2 min or so and it is untrue to say, as it so often is, that the 'immediate' nephrogram is due to filtered contrast. There is a significant blood-pool contribution to the early nephrogram.

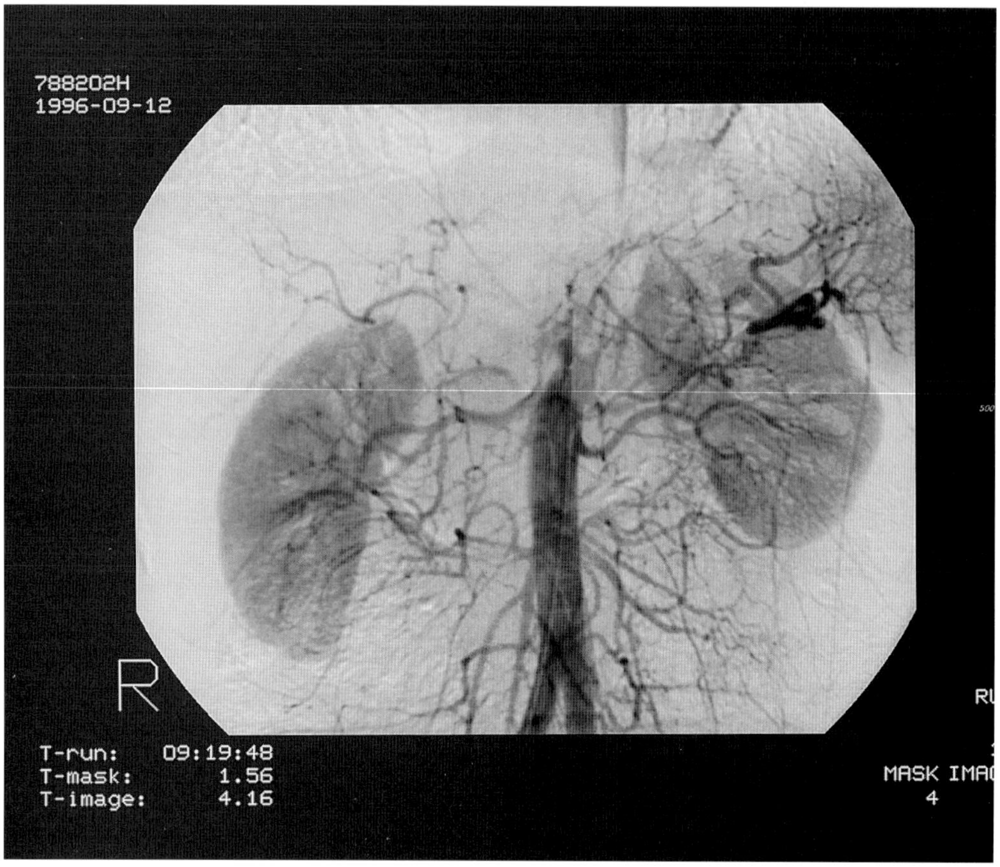

Figure 8.9
A digital immediate nephrogram.

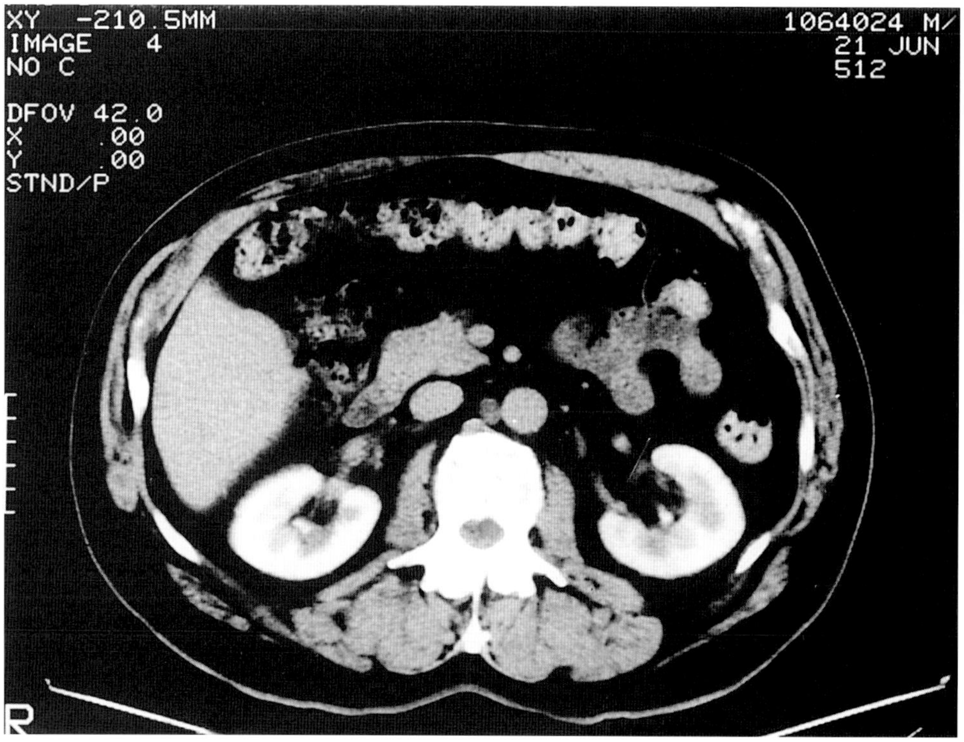

Figure 8.10
Persistent CT nephrograms 24 h after an arteriogram. Contrast-agent associated nephrotoxic event in a patient with pre-existing functional impairment.

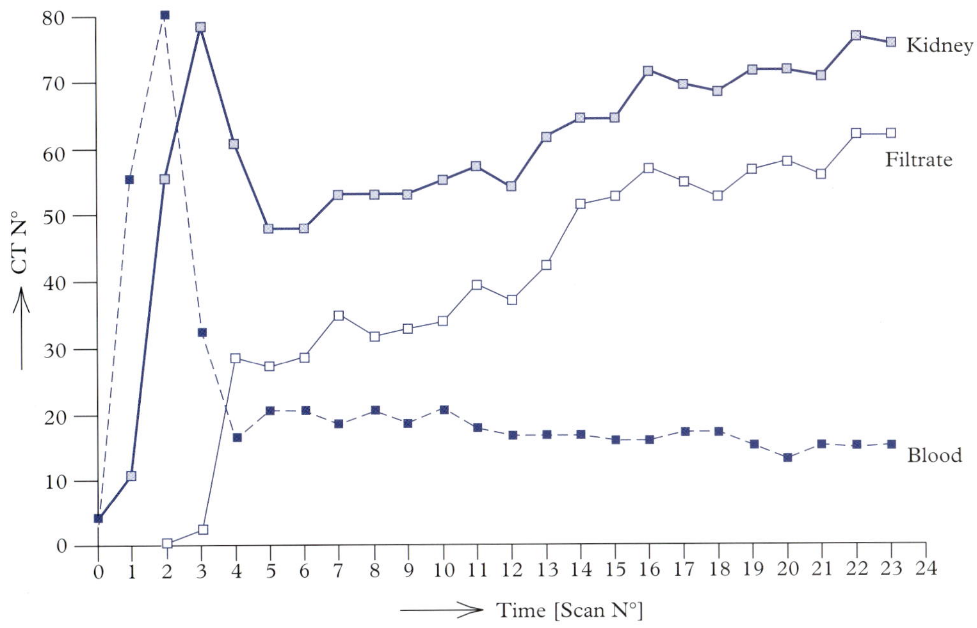

Figure 8.11
CT N° versus time curves for the whole kidney and for the aorta, scaled by a factor 0.3 to convert it to a renal blood-pool curve. The filtrate curve is obtained by subtraction. The relative contributions to the nephrogram of blood pool and filtered contrast at any time may be simply read off.

THE TRANSPLANT KIDNEY

A similar approach may be made to the transplant kidney. Here an iliac artery usually must be used as the arterial input curve, but the remainder of the technique and analysis remain much the same.

Figure 8.12 shows the results for a normally functioning transplant kidney and for a biopsy proven rejecting kidney. The reduced slope, indicating a reduced GFR, is an obvious and predictable finding. The reduced value of ϕ_b, the intercept on the ordinate, is much less predictable. It indicates a reduced proportionate vascular volume and may reasonably be interpreted as reflecting

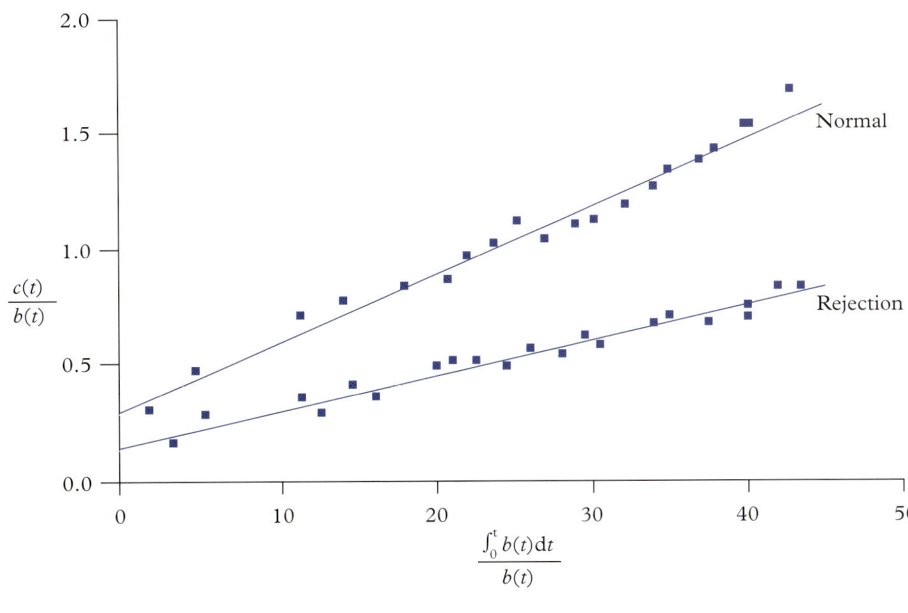

Figure 8.12
Patlak plots for normally functioning and rejecting transplant kidneys. Not only is the slope (GFR) reduced in the latter, but so is the ordinate intercept — the proportionate vascular volume. This may reflect small-vessel obliteration in the rejection process.

the obliteration of small vessels in severe rejection. While this remains to be confirmed in a large series of transplants, it may represent an approach to the non-invasive diagnosis of rejection and to its differentiation from other causes of renal-transplant function decline.

PHYSIOLOGICAL EFFECTS OF TRACER

The above procedures, like those for the assessment of perfusion, require the injection of 25 ml or so of contrast agent. X-ray contrast agents have a great variety of adverse effects on cardiac-pump function and electrophysiology [18] and on peripheral vasculature [19]. If a non-ionic agent is used, experience and monitoring indicate there is no significant change in systemic blood pressure associated with the injection and no significant change in heart rate. However, we know that contrast agents may have an effect on renal blood flow and consequently on GFR by a variety of other mechanisms [20–26] (Chapter 3). There is certainly an increase in circulating vasopressin levels within 1 min or so of injection. Injection of 50 ml of a non-ionic agent results in a doubling of circulating levels [23,24]; 25 ml would be expected to produce only a 50% rise since the effect is directly proportional to osmotic load. This is a small increase and is rather transient, falling back to baseline within a minute or so. The best evidence that there is no significant modification of blood flow (or presumably GFR) following injection of contrast in such a regime is that the values obtained for renal perfusion are so close to accepted values [9]. This gives considerable reason for confidence that there will be no significant modification of GFR during much the same regime.

PARAMETRIC IMAGING

We have seen in Chapters 6 and 7 how perfusion may be calculated on a pixel-by-pixel basis and the values colour-coded to generate parametric images. The same procedure may be carried out with the Patlak analysis and maps of the distribution of renal function through cortex and medulla thereby generated. Such a procedure might be helpful in indicating whether a renal disorder is a generalized or patchy process.

REFERENCES

1. Dawson, P. (1996) Glomerular filtration rate determined using contrast clearance: should we all be doing it? *Current Opinion in Urology*. In press.
2. Dawson, P. and Peters, A.M. (1993) Functional imaging in CT. The use of contrast enhanced CT for the study of renal function and physiology. *Investigative Radiology*, **28**, 579–584.
3. Dawson, P. and Peters, A.M. (1996) Renal function and the excretion of contrast agents. *British Journal of Radiology*, **69**, 567–569.

4. Dawson, P. and Blomley, M.J.K. (1996) Contrast media as extra-cellular fluid space markers: adaptation of the central volume theorem. *British Journal of Radiology*, **19**, 717–722.
5. Blomley, M.J.K. and Dawson, P. (1996) The quantification of renal function with computerised tomography. *British Journal of Radiology*, **69**, 989–995.
6. Dawson, P. and Peters, A.M. (1993) What is the nephrogram? *British Journal of Radiology*, **67**, 21–25.
7. Dawson, P. and Peters, A.M. (1993) Dynamic contrast bolus computerised tomography for the assessment of renal function. *Investigative Radiology*, **11**, 1039–1042.
8. Crone, C. and Levitt, D.G. (1987) Capillary permeability to small solutes. In *The Cardiovascular System*, Vol. IV, Part 1 (eds E.M. Renkin and C.C. Michell), pp. 411–466. Washington: American Physiological Society.
9. Blomley, M.J.K. and Dawson, P. (1993) Contrast bolus dynamic CT for the measurement of solid organ perfusion. *Investigative Radiology*, **28**, 572–577.
10. Blomley, M.J.K., Coulden, R., Dawson, P., Kormano, M., Donlan, P., Bufkin, C. and Lipton, M.J. (1997) Liver perfusion studies with ultrafast CT. *Academic Radiology*, *4(1)*, 13–20.
11. Blomley, M.J.K., Coulden, R., Kormano, M., Lim-Dunham, P., Dawson, P. and Lipton, M.J. (1997) Splenic blood flow; evaluation with CT. *Academic Radiology*, **4(1)**, 13–20.
12. Patlak, C.S., Blasberg, R.G. and Fenstermacher, J.D. (1983) Graphical evaluation of blood-to-brain barrier transfer constants from multiple time uptake data. *Cerebral Blood Flow and Metabolism*, **3**, 1–7.
13. Peters, A.M., George, P., Ballandie, F. *et al.* (1988) Appropriate selection of background for Tc-99m DTPA renography. *Nuclear Medicine Communications*, **9**, 973–985.
14. Peters, A.M. (1990) Measurement of microvascular permeability of small solutes in man. Limitations of the technique. *Cardiovascular Research*, **24**, 504–509.
15. Hillman, B., Lee, S.M., Tracey, P. *et al.* (1982) CT determination of renal and hepatic microvascular volumes in experimental acute renal failure. *Investigative Radiology*, **17**, 41–45.
16. Stewart, G.N. (1921) Tracer kinetics. *Journal of Physiology*, **50**, 20–37.
17. Kelsey-Fry, I. and Cattell, W.R. (1972) The nephrographic pattern during excretary urography. *British Medical Bulletin*, **28**, 227–232.
18. Hayward, R. and Dawson, P. (1984) Contrast agents in angiocardiography. *British Heart Journal*, **52**, 361–368.
19. Pugh, N.D., Sissons, G.R.J. and Ruttley, M.S.T. (1993) The effect of iodixanol, a new non-ionic contrast agent, on femoral blood flow in man. *Clinical Radiology*, **47**, 96–99.
20. Dawson, P. (1985) Contrast agent nephrotoxicity. An appraisal. *British Journal of Radiology*, **58**, 121–124.
21. Trewhella, M. and Dawson, P. (1990) Intravascular contrast agents and renal failure. *Clinical Radiology*, **41**, 373–375.
22. Dawson, P., Harrison, J.G. and Weisblatt, E. (1983) Effect of contrast media on red cell filtrability and morphology. *British Journal of Radiology*, **56**, 707–710.
23. Trewhella, M., Dawson, P., Rickards, D. and Forsling, M. (1987) Dehydration, ADH and the IVU. *British Journal of Radiology*, **60**, 445–447.
24. Trewhella, M., Forsling, M. and Dawson, P. (1990) Vasopressin release in response to intravenously injected contrast media. *British Journal of Radiology*, **63**, 97–100.

25. Strickland, N.S., Dawson, P., Rampling, M. and Martin, G. (1992) Contrast media induced effects on blood rheology and their importance in angiography. *Clinical Radiology*, **45**, 240–242.
26. Strickland, N.S., Dawson, P., Rampling, M. and Martin, G. (1992) The effects of radiocontrast media on rheological properties of blood. *Clinical Haemorheology*, **12**, 329–379.

Chapter 9
FUNCTIONAL CARDIAC CT

R. Coulden

The last thirty years have seen a revolution in medical imaging and nowhere is this more apparent than in the investigation of heart disease. Ischaemic heart disease is the commonest cause of death in the Western world and vast resources are consumed in its investigation and management. For most clinicians, the important questions concern coronary anatomy, myocardial perfusion and left-ventricular function. Coronary angiography provides exquisite anatomical detail of the epicardial vessels but gives no indication of the perfusion abnormality that results from a stenosis or occlusion. Radionuclide-perfusion imaging will show areas of relative myocardial hypoperfusion but, without quantification, assessment of their significance may be difficult. Absolute perfusion can be measured with positron emission tomography (PET) but technical problems, high cost and limited access make it an impractical clinical tool. Alternative methods for measuring myocardial perfusion are required. Echocardiography and angiography provide qualitative assessments of left-ventricular function but quantitation is unreliable. Both assume a specific geometry for ventricular shape which breaks down when the ventricle becomes dilated or asymmetric. Radionuclide ventriculography makes no assumptions and provides accurate, reproducible estimations of ejection fraction but there is no simple, broadly accepted approach to the measurement of stroke volume, cardiac output or regional wall motion [1]. Alternative methods for absolute quantification are required.

Functional computed tomography (CT) has been available in various guises for many years; however, long image-acquisition times and motion artefact have always prevented its use in the heart. To quantify ventricular function or myocardial perfusion, image-acquisition must be short enough to freeze cardiac motion and times of the order of tens of milliseconds are required. This was first achieved commercially by Boyd and his associates [2] in the early 1980s using an electron beam CT (EBCT) scanner capable of exposing a slice in 50 ms (C100, Imatron, San Francisco, USA). Over the last 15 years there have been numerous improvements in specification with the most recent developments made in conjunction with Siemens (Evolution XP, Siemens, Ehrlangen, Germany). There are now approximately 50 EBCT scanners worldwide and their use in the functional assessment of the heart is reviewed.

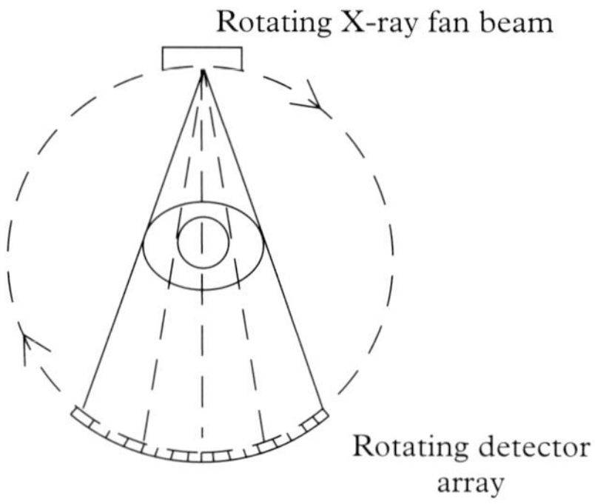

Generation III

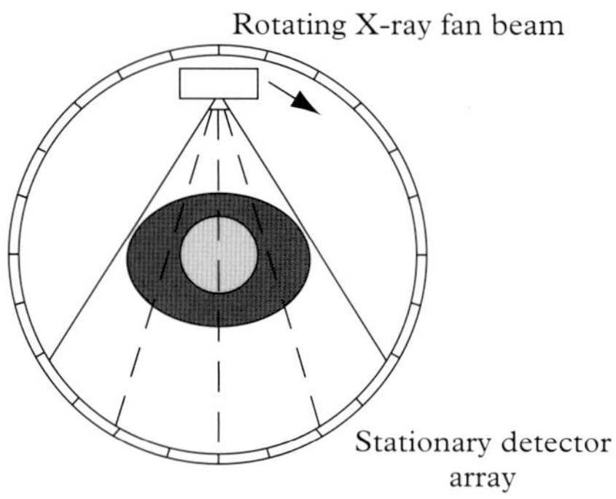

Generation IV

Figure 9.1
Diagrammatic representation of X-ray tube detector geometries for current third- and fourth-generation CT systems.

ELECTRON BEAM CT: TECHNICAL CONSIDERATIONS

Design and modes of operation

Electron beam CT differs fundamentally from conventional third- or fourth-generation scanners. With conventional CT, the X-ray tube and detector array rotate around the patient (third generation) or the X-ray tube rotates with a continuous ring of detectors remaining stationary around the patient (fourth generation) (Figure 9.1). These geometries, combined with the latest slip-ring technology, can give acquisition times as short as 0.75 s per slice (Somaton Plus 4, Siemens, Ehrlangen, Germany). However, this is still too long for cardiac imaging. Continued development is likely but the huge mass of the X-ray tube and its detector assembly (approximately 1 tonne) will make additional reductions in image time difficult to achieve and prohibitively expensive.

The EBCT scanner is the first fifth-generation scanner and has a completely different geometry to its predecessors. The X-ray target is a 210° tungsten arc that partly encloses the patient posteriorly. The detector array covers a similar arc anteriorly (Figure 9.2). An image is produced by sweeping a tightly focused 130 kV electron beam across the tungsten target over a period of 50 ms. There

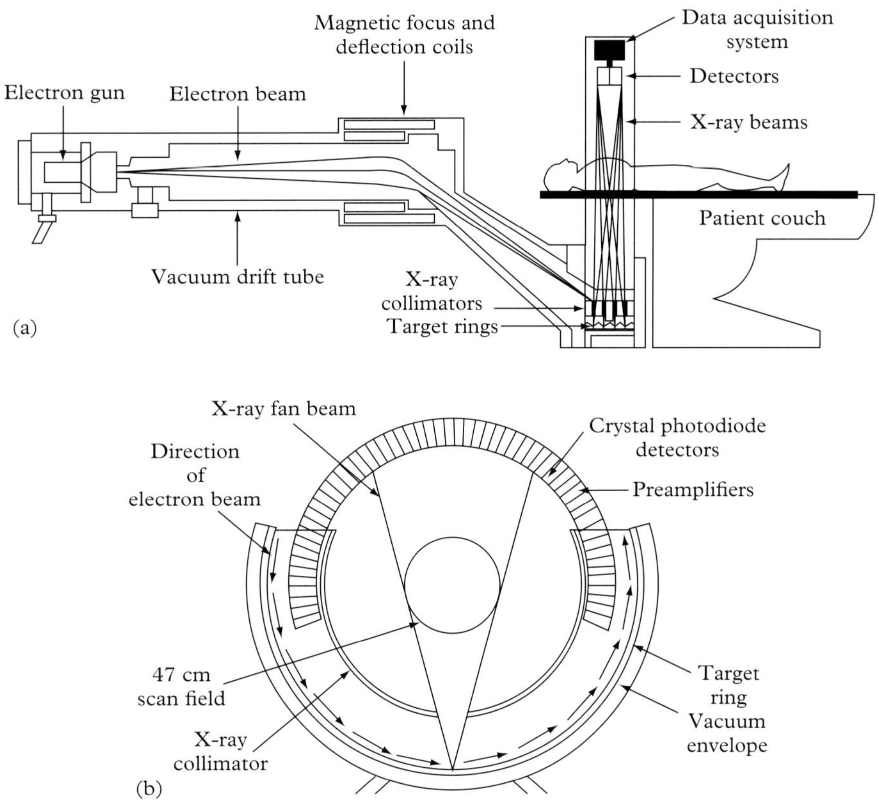

Figure 9.2
(a) Longitudinal section through an EBCT system showing the electron gun and the magnetic focus and deflection coils which sweep the electron beam across the four tungsten target rings. Collimated X-rays from each target ring are detected by a pair of contiguous detector arrays allowing up to eight slices to be acquired without moving the patient couch. (b) Transverse section at the level of the target rings shows that each ring is incomplete and covers a 210° arc below the patient. An opposing and partly overlapping arc of detectors collects data from the fan of X-rays generated as the electron beam is swept across each target ring. (Reproduced with permission from D.P. Boyd, R.G. Gould, J.R. Quinn, *et al.* (1979) A proposed dynamic cardiac 3-D densitometer for early detection and evaluation of heart disease. *IEEE Transactions on Nuclear Science*, **26**, 2724.)

are no moving parts. To improve patient coverage in the *z*-axis, four target rings are included within the vacuum envelope and there are two detector arrays. With this arrangement, each target ring can be used in turn to generate two contiguous slices giving up to eight slice levels without moving the patient. Slice thickness can be varied from 1.5 to 10 mm and target sweep times can be varied from 50 to 100 ms. In the single-slice mode, data from multiple sweeps of a single target ring can be summed to reduce noise and improve image quality but this is always at the expense of increased scan time (maximum summed scan time, 2 s). With a short acquisition time and very high heat capacity, EBCT is ideally suited to continuous volume scanning. However, the unusual geometry creates gaps in the resulting data helix and reconstruction is complex. New reconstruction algorithms have solved this problem and it is now possible to acquire up to 126 slices in 15 s (Evolution XP, Siemens, Ehrlangen, Germany). In the single-slice mode up to 40 levels can be obtained, the exact time taken depending on slice thickness, table movement and exposure time.

For cardiac imaging, three scan modes are available: ECG-triggered single slice mode, cine mode and flow mode (Figure 9.3). In the standard single-slice mode, only one target ring is used with table increments after each acquisition. The short acquisition time of 50 ms or 100 ms prevents motion artefact but cardiac motion can still cause misregistration between slices, particularly when slices are thin. ECG triggering overcomes this and is most effective when used in mid-diastole (the 'quiet' period of the cardiac cycle). This is achieved by applying

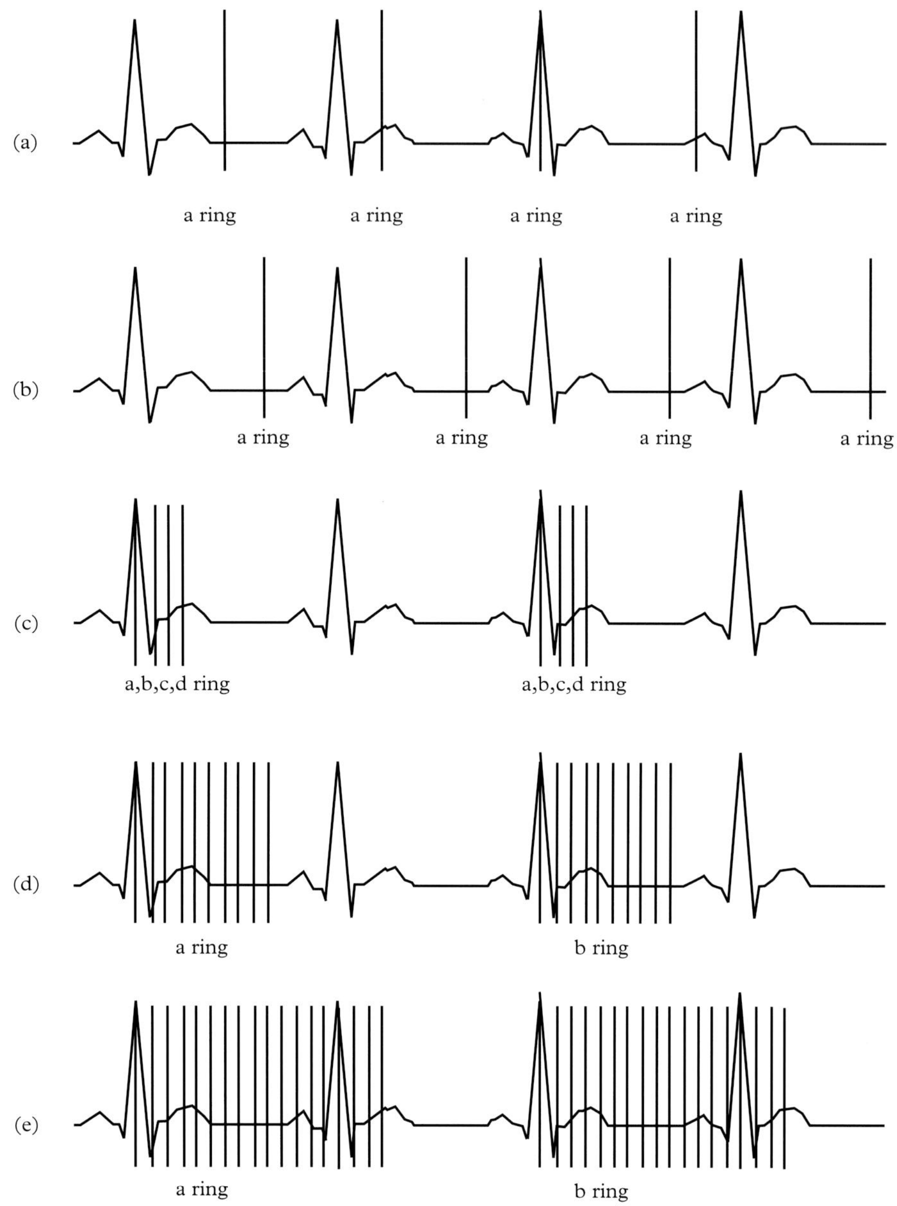

Figure 9.3
Rapid-image acquisition and choice of four target rings gives a range of imaging options. In the single-slice mode (a), one target ring is used with or without table motion and each slice is acquired at a different point in the cardiac cycle. With cardiac triggering, repeated image acquisition at one level gives a series of images over time in the same phase of the cardiac cycle (b). This mode is ideally suited to tracking a bolus of intravenous contrast medium through cardiac chambers and myocardium. Using all four target rings and a cardiac trigger, up to eight levels can be acquired in the same phase of the cardiac cycle over time (c). This allows bolus tracking within a volume of tissue. Data acquisition can be triggered to occur on every cycle or alternate cycles depending on heart rate and rate of contrast transit. Rapid continuous image acquisition (one image every 58 ms) using the same target ring creates a cine sequence at one level (d). By using different rings with each beat up to eight contiguous levels can be obtained. Volume cine data of this sort is used for assessment of cardiac function. If diastolic function is to be assessed, image acquisition must extend beyond one R–R interval and the cardiac trigger must be on alternate beats (e).

a delay after the R-wave trigger equivalent to 80% of the R–R interval. In the cine mode, the same target ring is exposed repeatedly every 58 ms following the R wave, i.e. multiple images at a single level or pair of levels during a single cardiac cycle. After a predetermined number of exposures, there is a pause until the next R wave when the process is repeated using the next target ring. In this way, up to eight sets of cine images can be obtained at eight contiguous levels during seven heartbeats. The acquisition is not gated as in magnetic resonance imaging (MRI) or radionuclide ventriculography because a complete cine dataset is obtained in a single heartbeat. It is not the composite of many beats. In the flow mode, each of the target rings is swept in turn after a trigger from the R wave of the ECG. This is then repeated on every beat or on alternate beats giving rise to a series of scans over time at up to eight levels. The scan series for each level is at the same point in the cardiac cycle, ensuring accurate slice-to-slice registration for time–density measurements. Time delays after the R-wave trigger can be applied as with other modes to give datasets at any point in the cardiac cycle.

The wide gantry aperture permitted by EBCT geometry allows the patient couch to tilt and swivel (swivel to right or left 25°, downward tilt 23°). This is particularly useful for cardiac studies as it enables imaging in the short or long axis of the left ventricle, aiding functional assessment.

Performance

EBCT clearly has great advantages over conventional CT for cardiac imaging but the very short acquisition times and asymmetric geometry have their penalties. Distribution of patient radiation dose through the slice is asymmetric when compared with conventional CT (Figure 9.4) and this together with a low

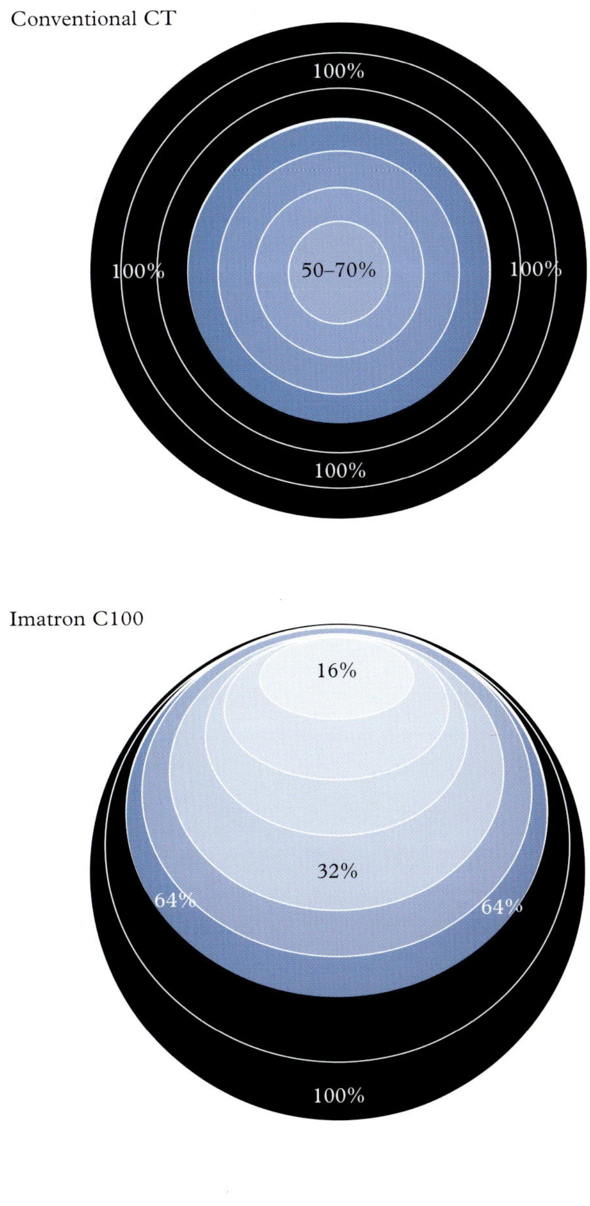

Figure 9.4
Radiation dose distribution within a 32 cm homogeneous phantom. With conventional CT, the maximum dose is deposited in the periphery of the object and is distributed evenly around the perimeter. Dose distribution with EBCT, however, is asymmetric with the greatest radiation dose inferiorly and a reduction in dose towards the top.

Scanner	Noise σ (HU)	Spatial resolution (lp/cm)	Contrast resolution (mm)	Uniformity (%)
Imatron C100	19	5	4.5	12
GE 9800	16	6.25	4	4

Noise is the random fluctuation of CT numbers in a uniform object and is measured as the standard deviation of pixel values located within a region of interest at the centre of the object. Spatial resolution refers to the number of high-contrast line pairs that can be resolved in 1 cm in a homogeneous field. Contrast resolution indicates the smallest object in mm, differing from its background by 6 HU, that can be identified in a uniform field. Uniformity is defined as the percentage difference in CT number between the centre and edge of a homogeneous field. (Values based on C.H. McCollough and R.L. Morin (1994) The technical design and performance of ultrafast computed tomography. *Radiology Clinics of North America*, **32**, 521–536.)

Table 9.1
Comparison of Imatron C100 and GE 9800 scanners

exposure per slice (32 mAs or 64 mAs for a 50 ms or 100 ms acquisition, respectively) exacerbates image noise. Spatial resolution is theoretically independent of radiation exposure, but will be impaired when noise is significant. Contrast resolution, however, is strongly influenced by radiation exposure. Short acquisition times with a low exposure mean poorer contrast resolution compared with conventional CT. Image uniformity refers to the uniformity of Hounsfield number across the reconstructed field of view. Corrections are made by the reconstruction algorithm to minimize variations in mean Hounsfield number between the centre and edge of the field of view but when the imaged object has a heterogeneous attenuation, this correction may be inadequate. Table 9.1 compares noise, spatial resolution, contrast resolution and image uniformity between EBCT (Imatron C100, 8 mm slice thickness and 0.05 s data acquisition) and a conventional CT system (GE 9800, 10 mm slice thickness and 2 s data acquisition) [3].

Software tools are available to measure distance and area within the slice plane and accuracy for conventional CT and EBCT is similar. Slice width, however, is not uniform across the field of view with EBCT because the target and detector rings are not in the same plane. The X-ray beam maps out a conical volume through the patient resulting in an increase in slice width at the periphery. This is important when measuring small objects or objects with a radius of curvature similar to the slice thickness. They should be placed at the centre of the field of view rather than at the edge.

VENTRICULAR FUNCTION

The high temporal and spatial resolution of EBCT are ideally suited to the accurate assessment of cardiac motion. For most purposes, this means ventricular function and wall motion but the techniques apply equally well to the atria. The use of ECG triggering rather than gating also confers advantages over competing techniques like radionuclide ventriculography or MRI.

Data acquisition

Measurement of ventricular function is performed in the short axis of the left ventricle (table swivelled 25° to the patient's right and tilted down 20°) during an intravenous bolus of contrast medium. The cine mode is used, with the number of images per level being adjusted to cover the whole of systole. If diastolic function is also going to be assessed, the number of images per level must be increased to extend beyond the next R wave of the ECG (Figure 9.3). In this way, up to eight cine slices covering 8 cm in the z-axis can be acquired during a single contrast bolus. With such a short acquisition protocol (seven heartbeats), timing of the acquisition to the intravenous contrast bolus is essential and some means of measuring circulation time is required. This can be done using indocyanin green and an ear oximeter [4], injecting intravenous magnesium sulphate and timing the delay to the patient experiencing a salty taste in the mouth or simply measuring the time taken for a test bolus of contrast to reach the left heart by repeated CT scanning at one level [5]. To minimize motion artefact, all images are acquired in suspended respiration and rarely take more than 10 s per dataset. Non-ionic contrast medium is used to reduce the haemodynamic consequences of contrast administration, i.e. transient tachycardia, rise in blood pressure, increase in stroke volume (see Chapter 3), and to improve the validity of the measurement [6]. In patients with poor ventricular function and long circulation times, faster rates of contrast administration are usually needed (contrast injection rate increased from 2 to 2.5 or 3 ml/s). These patients may also have cardiomegaly and need two contiguous 8 cm volume datasets to cover the whole ventricle, each one necessitating a separate contrast bolus.

Image analysis and edge detection

All measurements of ventricular function and mass derived from cine data, be it EBCT or MRI, require identification of the endocardial and epicardial borders. This is usually done by hand but as with all operator-intensive analysis is subject to errors. One of the most important relates to the displayed window level and width (Figure 9.5). Feiring *et al.* [7] found that myocardial mass best correlated with postmortem results in dogs, when the image to be analysed displayed the whole range of attenuation values across a boundary. The true boundary lay at an attenuation number 'half-way' between the mean attenuation values of the two boundary structures (threshold value). For practical purposes, this amounts to setting the window level at the threshold value and the width at twice the threshold. Where adjacent structures are heterogeneous, the threshold value may vary along the border, making it necessary to set different window levels and widths at multiple points.

(a)

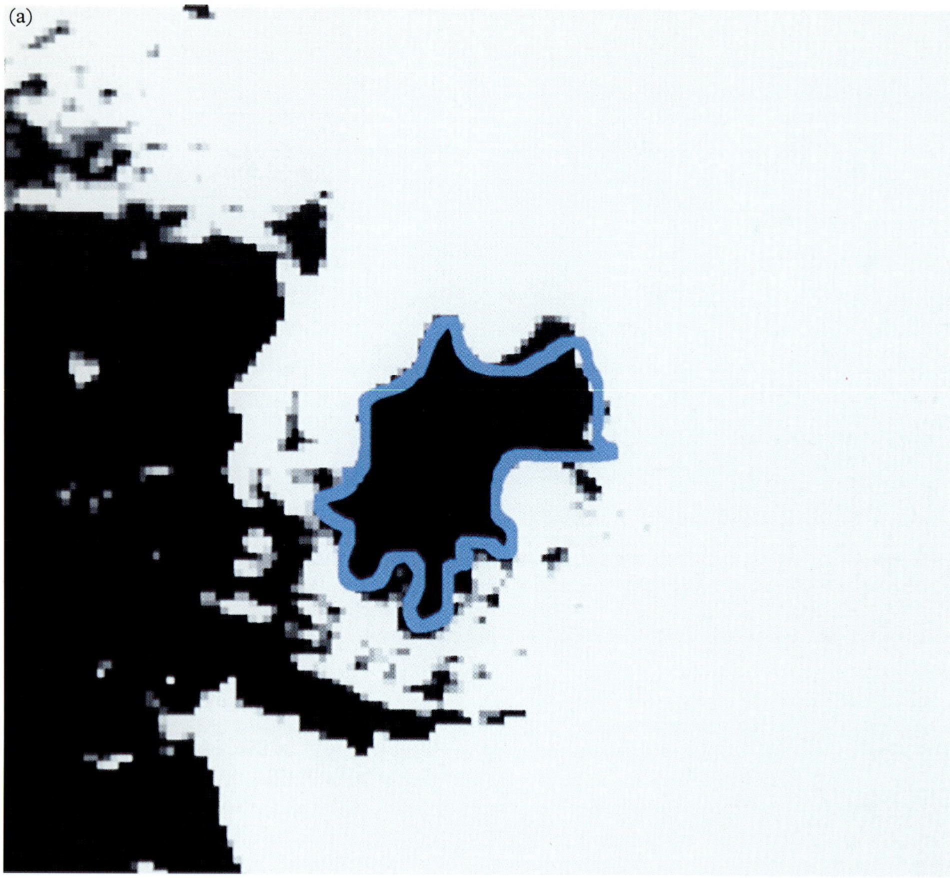

(b)

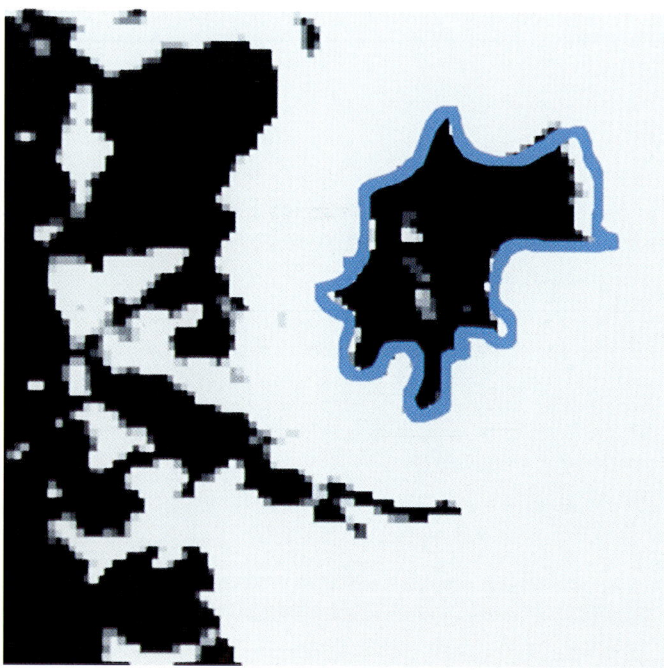

Figure 9.5
Window level is an important variable when defining the position of the endocardial border. All three views of the short axis of the left ventricle have the same endocardial boundary outlined in grey but as the window level is altered [(a) = 75 HU, (b) = 95 HU, (c) = 115 HU)] the apparent cavity dimensions can be artificially increased or decreased. Window width has been fixed at 2 making these binary images.

Figure 9.5
(continued)

(c)

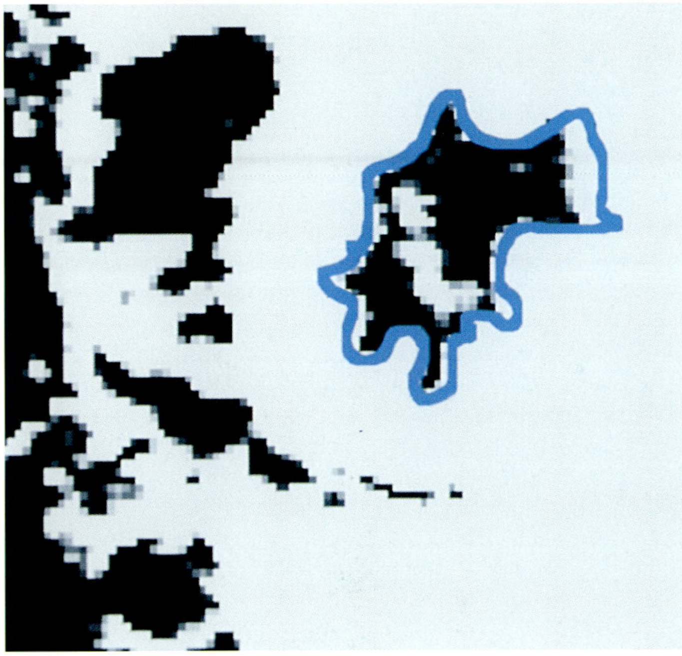

Such an approach improves inter- and intra-observer variability but manual analysis is far too time consuming for non-research use. A rapid and robust automated method is urgently required. Several have been described but no one method has gained general acceptance, as evidenced by the lack of commercial software for ventricular analysis. Postprocessing algorithms fall into three main categories: edge tracking, segmentation and stereology.

Edge tracking

Edge tracking is widely available and in its simplest form tracks the boundary from a seed border pixel which has been identified manually [8]. The method is effective when signal-to-noise ratios are high but founders when boundaries are indistinct. It is also highly dependent on the operator's choice of border pixel. Filtering may help to enhance edges prior to tracking but improved tracking is offset by difficulties in ensuring that the edge that is enhanced is genuinely at the boundary. Great care must be taken to tailor the specific filter to the type of image and boundary being analysed. More sophisticated algorithms using dynamic programming and graph searching have been described for MRI data but they have yet to be used for CT [9,10]. By predefining the shape of the left ventricle, i.e. radial symmetry, the tracking algorithm can be constrained to improve reliability [11,12]. However, it is then dogged by the same inaccuracies as standard two-dimensional techniques when faced with a diseased or asymmetric ventricle.

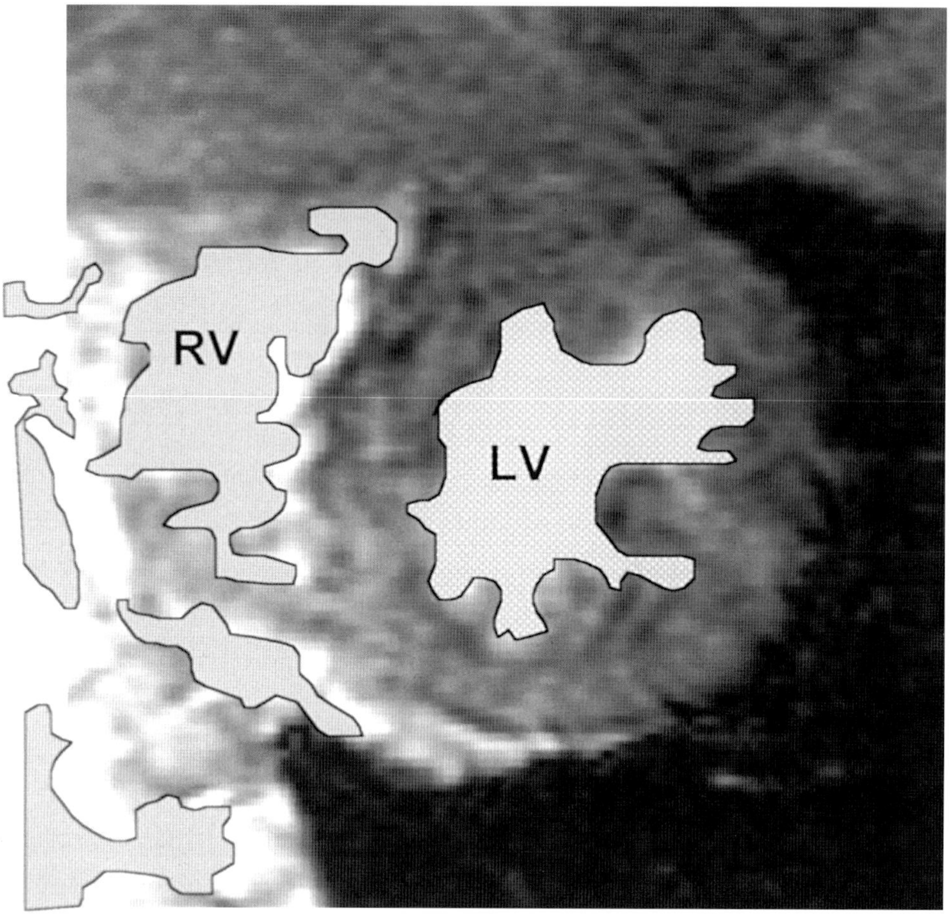

Figure 9.6
On this short-axis image of the left ventricle, all areas above a threshold attenuation value have been outlined in grey. In order to separate right- and left-ventricular cavities, only those voxels in continuity with a seed voxel in the left-ventricular blood pool are included (grey hatch). Connectivity is a three-dimensional process and extends to slices above and below, creating a volume of contiguous voxels.

Segmentation

Segmentation provides an alternative approach and is generally more robust when applied to low signal-to-noise ratio images. The boundary is defined automatically as the edge of a selected region of interest (ROI) whose pixels fulfil specific criteria. The most basic form of segmentation involves thresholding and connectivity. Considering the left-ventricular blood pool during contrast enhancement, a threshold is chosen which identifies all pixels with a value equal to, or greater than, contrast-enhanced blood. This highlights pixels in both left- and right-ventricular blood pools. To define the left-ventricular cavity as separate from the right, a seed is then placed in the left-ventricular blood pool and only those pixels in continuity with it are included. The right-ventricular blood pool, separated from the left by a low attenuation ventricular septum is discarded (Figure 9.6). Choice of threshold is again crucial; too high a threshold and the segmented area will be smaller than expected, too low and it will be larger. To reduce variability, but not necessarily improve accuracy, the threshold can be determined automatically. Class variance has been widely used with other modalities for image postprocessing and can be applied here. A histogram of attenuation values is derived from a ROI which includes both sides of the boundary. This gives two populations of pixels, each representing one side of the

(a) (b)

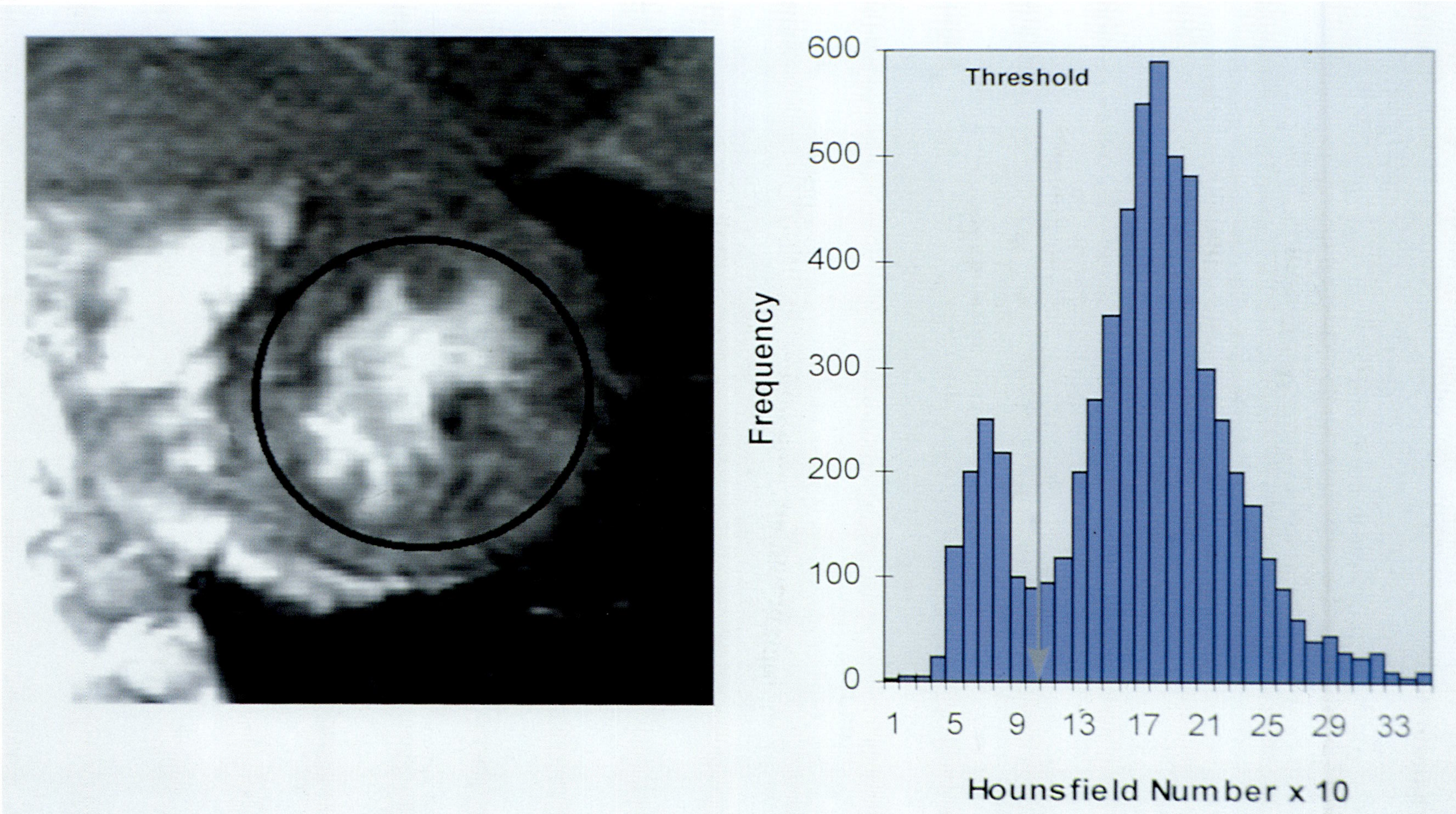

Figure 9.7
(a) Short-axis view of the left ventricle with a circular region of interest (ROI) applied. (b) Class variance uses a histogram of all pixel values within a ROI to identify the most appropriate threshold for detecting the endocardial border. When the ROI contains two populations of pixel values (myocardium and blood pool), the threshold is defined as the minimum value between the two peaks.

boundary. The attenuation value with minimum incidence between the two peaks is the optimum threshold (Figure 9.7). Unfortunately, this too has its drawbacks. A single threshold is not ideal and algorithms that search for boundaries using peak rate of change of attenuation number may be more appropriate. Additional constraints, such as boundary smoothing or *a priori* knowledge of ventricular shape, are also being considered.

These methods are increasingly successful at defining the blood pool within the body of the left ventricle but identification of the valve plane on a short-axis image remains difficult. Cardiac long-axis views can be reconstructed from short-axis datasets and this has been used to define valve plane on MRI images [13]. The same technique should be applicable to the EBCT data but has yet to be tried.

Stereology

Stereology differs from the other methods in that it is neither automatic nor boundary-defining. It is, however, considerably faster than simple manual edge detection. The observer defines the ROI by deleting all points that lie within it

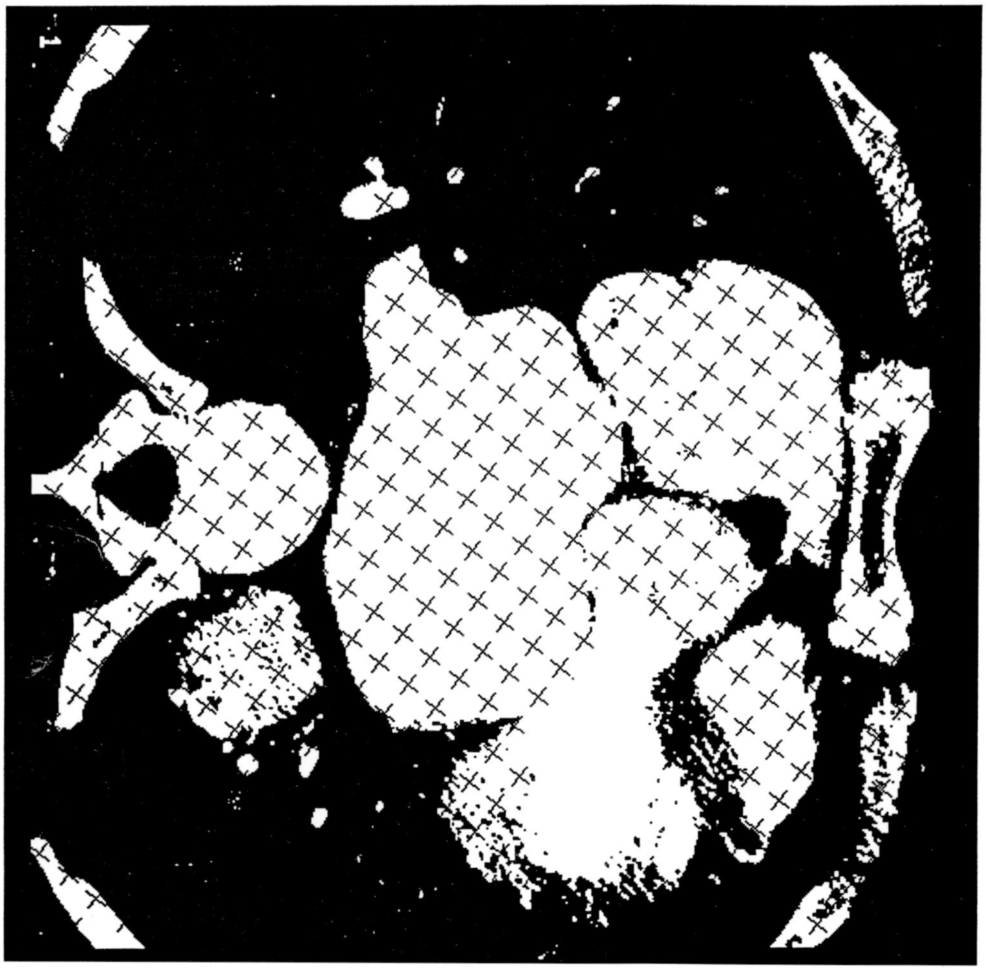

Figure 9.8
Image from a cine sequence of the left ventricle with a random grid of crosses applied. Stereology requires the observer to identify all crosses within the region of interest, i.e. the blood pool, and to repeat the process for all images making up to the volume at the same phase of the cardiac cycle. By summing all identified crosses, ventricular volume can be calculated and an estimate of error made.

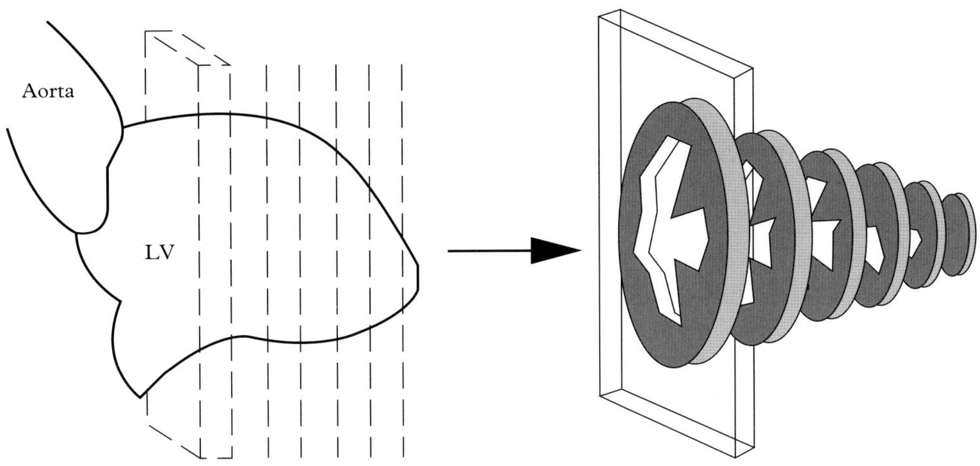

Figure 9.9
Calculation of left-ventricular volume from the cross-sectional areas of the blood pool within adjacent slices at the same phase of the cardiac cycle. Volume equals summed area multiplied by slice thickness (Simpson's rule). No geometric assumptions are made.

from a grid that has been applied randomly to the image (Figure 9.8) [14]. The number of points deleted as a proportion of total points in the field of view is then used to calculate cross-sectional area. Unlike the other methods, the measured area has a statistical basis and an estimate of the error is provided.

Indices of ventricular function

Once endocardial and epicardial borders are defined, standard parameters of ventricular function can be derived using Simpson's rule (Figure 9.9). There is no assumption of ventricular shape, as is required by echocardiography or angiography, and the approach is accurate even in the presence of regional wall motion abnormalities. The observer selects end-diastolic and end-systolic images from each cine dataset, sums the areas of the segmented blood pool for all levels and multiplies by slice thickness, calculates end-diastolic volume, end-systolic volume, stroke volume, ejection fraction and cardiac output.* The only difficulty lies in selecting the end-systolic frame and this is best done using the time delay for aortic valve closure as determined on the cine loop of the aortic root. The accuracy of EBCT is now well established and several reports have validated the technique for both right and left ventricles (Figure 9.10) [15–17]. For the right ventricle, this is a particular advantage as there is no satisfactory geometric model for use with echocardiography or angiography. EBCT or MRI are now the modalities of choice for investigating the right heart. In healthy individuals the stroke volumes of right and left ventricles are virtually identical, small differences being due to physiological shunts, i.e. bronchial blood flow. In patients with an incompetent valve, comparison of right- and left-ventricular stroke volumes has been shown to be accurate in quantifying regurgitant fraction, an important determinant in the timing of surgical correction [18].

---

*Stroke volume (SV) = end-diastolic volume (EDV) – end-systolic volume (ESV). Ejection fraction = SV/EDV, Cardiac output = SV × heart rate.

(a)

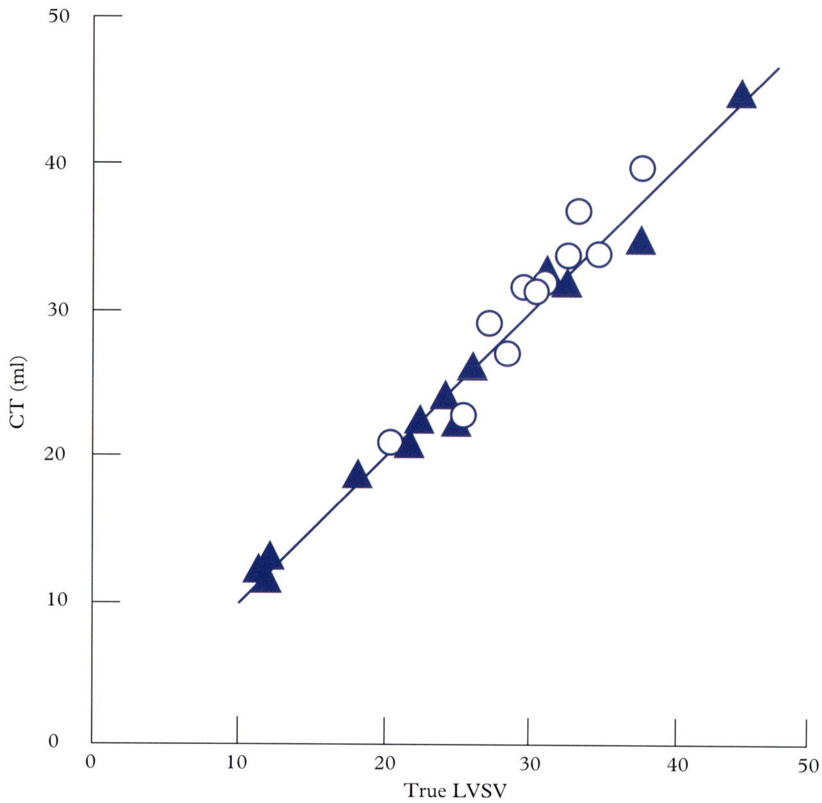

Figure 9.10
(a) Comparison of global left-ventricular function measured by EBCT with estimates made using thermodilution (▲) or implanted electromagnetic aortic flow (O) meter (EMF) in dogs. $n = 25$; $r = 0.99$; y-intercept = –0.24 ml; slope = 1.01; SEE = 1.47 ml. (b) Same methodology used for the right ventricle. $n = 15$; $r = 0.98$; y-intercept = 2.22 ml; slope = 0.89; SEE = 1.73 ml. (Reproduced with permission from S.J. Reiter, J.A. Rumberger, A.J. Feiring *et al.* (1986) Precision of right- and left-ventricular stroke volume measurements by rapid acquisition cine-computed tomography. *Circulation*, **74**, 890–900.)

(b)

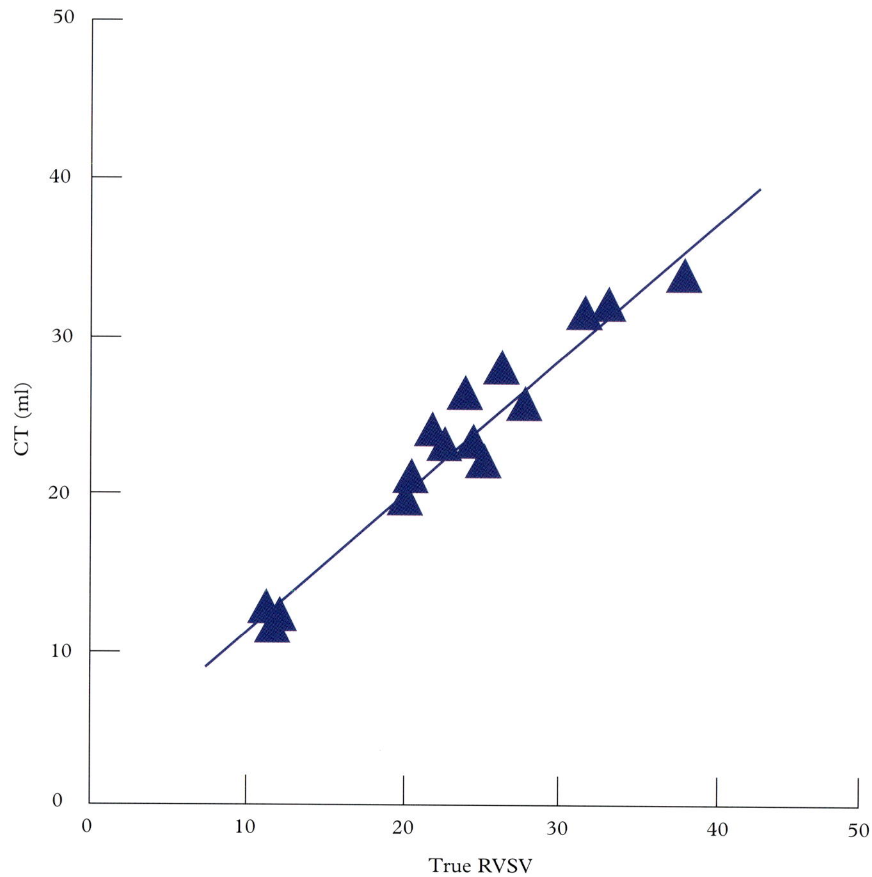

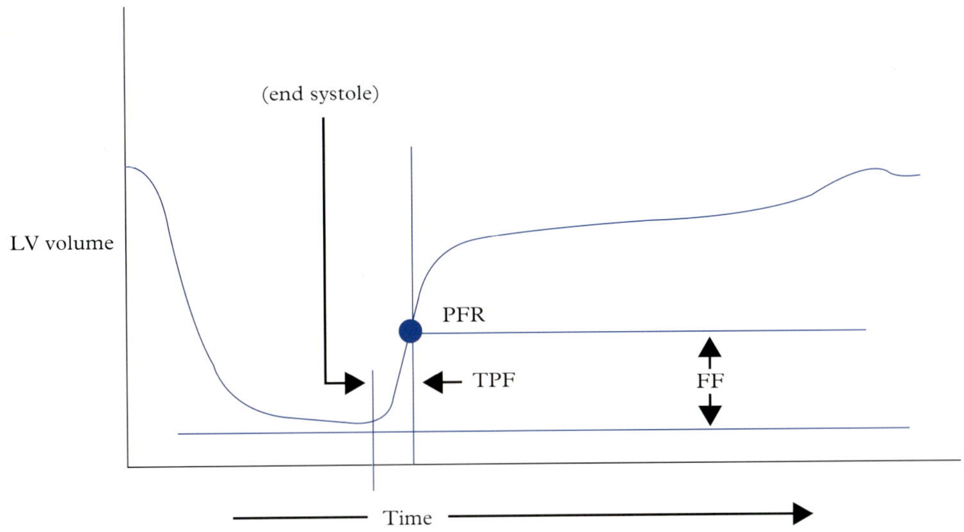

Figure 9.11
Graphical representation of left-ventricular (LV) volume with time as derived from a cine CT dataset of the left ventricle. Peak flow rate (PFR) and time to peak flow (TPF) are important parameters in assessing diastolic function. Filling fraction (FF), the percentage of total diastolic filling that has recurred by TPF, has also been found to be an indicator of ventricular compliance. (Reproduced with permission from J.A. Rumberger (1992) Use of ultrafast computed tomography to assess early diastolic filling in man. In: *Ultrafast Computed Tomography in Cardiac Imaging* W. Stanford and J.A. Rumberger (eds). Mount Kisko, NY: Futura. pp. 161–175.

By calculating ventricular volumes at multiple time points throughout the cardiac cycle, time–volume curves can be created for both left and right ventricles (Figure 9.11). Such curves correlate well with radionuclide ventriculography and are a useful alternative to Doppler and M-mode echocardiography for assessing global diastolic function [19]. Unlike conventional radionuclide ventriculography, however, EBCT provides a way of interrogating regional diastolic function in three dimensions. Investigating the left ventricle, Rumberger *et al.* [20] confirmed the intimate relationship between regional rates of diastolic filling and regional ventricular size, peak filling rates being greater at the apex than the base. Similar results were obtained for the right ventricle, but as the volume of the normal right ventricle is larger than the left, filling rates as a proportion of end-diastolic volume were lower [21]. Peak filling rates are an important indicator of ventricular compliance and in ischaemic heart disease may be abnormal before there is evidence of systolic dysfunction. Accurate measurement of peak filling rate requires multiple data points on the up-slope of the curve. When diastole is shortened, i.e. heart rates above 90 bpm, the maximum frame rate of EBCT (17 fps) may be insufficient.

As with ventricular volumes, the volume of myocardial muscle can be obtained by planimetry of epicardial and endocardial surfaces and applying Simpson's rule. To calculate mass, a simple correction is made to allow for the density of myocardial muscle (1.05 g/cm^3). The mass of both right and left ventricles, validated by several authors, has been shown to have excellent reproducibility [22,23]. A significant proportion of myocardial volume is vascular and this, of course, changes between systole and diastole. In systole, when intramural pressure is high and perfusion low, vascular volume is reduced and vice versa. Diastolic estimates of myocardial mass correlate best with the mass observed from postmortem specimens and are generally used.

Global ventricular function and mass measurements are clearly important but abnormalities frequently have to be severe to be detected. Ischaemic heart disease is a focal process and the cine dataset for each level provides the

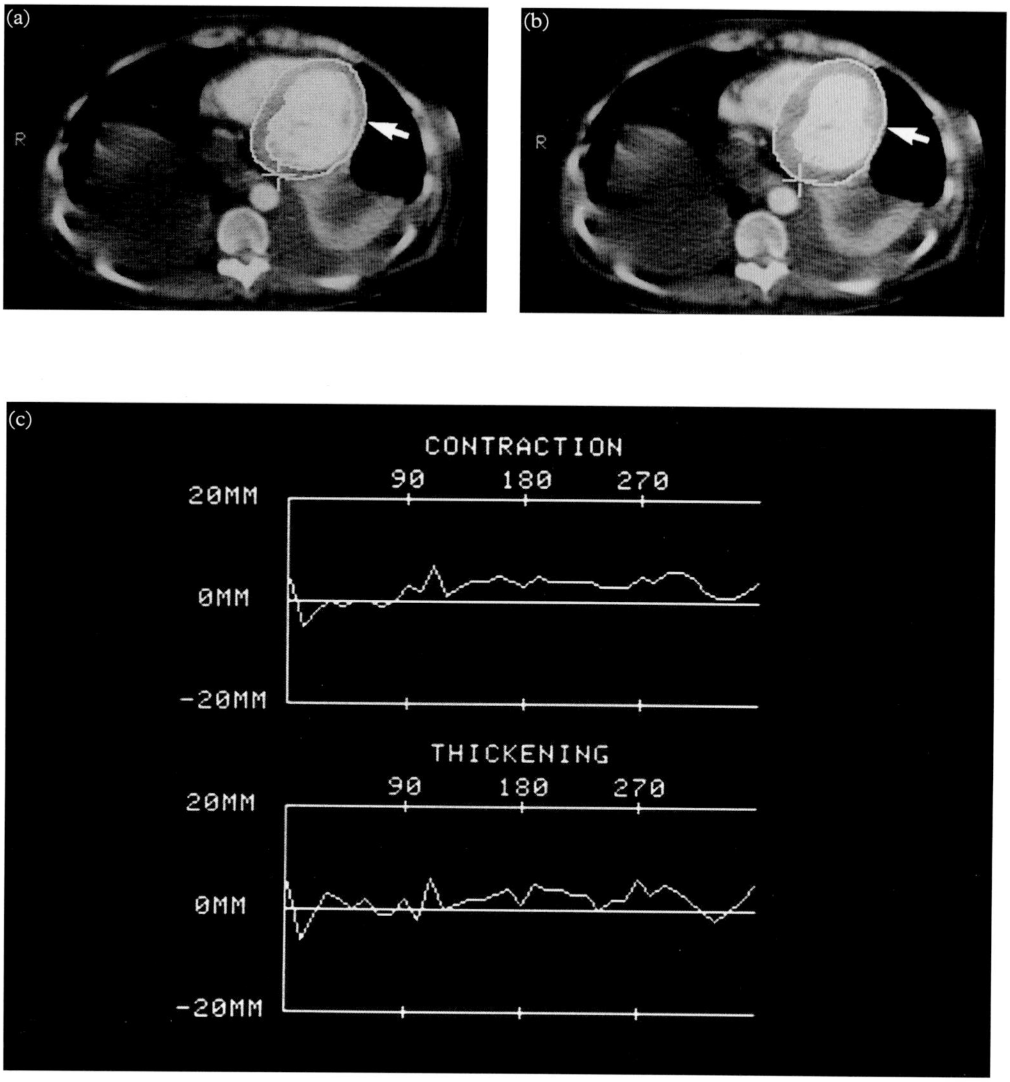

Figure 9.12
Endocardial and epicardial boundaries define left-ventricular muscle mass in diastole (a) and systole (b) in this patient with infarction of the free wall of the left ventricle (arrows). Change in boundary position between the two images is then used to calculate contraction and wall thickening (c). Absence of thickening and contraction along the free wall of the ventricle. (0–90°) corresponds to the site of infarction.

opportunity to look for regional abnormalities. Once endocardial and epicardial boundaries have been defined, wall motion can be examined in terms of phase, amplitude of excursion and wall thickening (Figure 9.12). By repeating the examination after stress, which can be pharmacological or physical, it is possible to screen for myocardial ischaemia. This may be reflected as a failure to increase stroke volume by more than 5% or as a focal abnormality of wall motion. The capacity of EBCT to characterize wall motion has already been exploited by Lessick *et al.* [24] who used the technique to examine post-infarction aneurysms prior to surgery. They showed that, in many cases, the thinned aneurysmal scar was surrounded by a penumbra of myocardium of normal thickness but impaired function. While the reason for the penumbra was unclear (probably due to abnormal wall stress, chronic ischaemia or both), the study did show that its extent was a useful predictor of outcome following aneurysmectomy. Low-dose dobutamine infusion has been used in conjunction with echocardiography to detect hibernating myocardium but analysis was always hampered by poor quantification. EBCT with its clearer border definition and range of quantitative analysis tools makes an ideal alternative but this has yet to be confirmed.

BLOOD FLOW AND MYOCARDIAL PERFUSION

The measurement of myocardial perfusion has long been seen as the 'Holy Grail' of cardiac imaging. Radionuclide perfusion methods provide a qualitative guide to perfusion but this is often difficult to correlate with sites of coronary stenosis when disease is extensive [25]. Non-invasive measurements of tissue perfusion and coronary artery flow reserve are required. The latter can be obtained using intracoronary Doppler ultrasound but difficulties establishing a reliable resting flow in this invasive setting can invalidate the measurement. EBCT has promised much over the years, yet has still to deliver. More success has been achieved, however, using time–attenuation curves during a bolus of contrast medium to measure large-vessel blood flow and cardiac shunts.

Data acquisition

Myocardial perfusion measurements are performed in the short axis of the left ventricle, while estimates of shunt fraction in congenital heart disease usually require the horizontal long axis (table swivelled 25° to patient's left, no tilt). For flow in large vessels, images should be obtained at right angles to the direction of flow. All images are acquired in the flow mode during a bolus of intravenous contrast medium. To prevent misregistration on time–attenuation analyses, examinations are performed during a breath-hold and acquisition is timed to produce the first image before contrast medium enters the right heart. Flow measurements are usually made in systole with up to four of the target rings being exposed in turn. Systolic images are chosen when measuring myocardial perfusion as they provide the greatest thickness of myocardial muscle for ROI analysis. End-systole can be obtained by applying an arbitrary 40% R–R interval delay to the R-wave trigger. Repeat measurements are made on each beat or on alternate beats for 20 s. The contrast bolus needs to be as compact as possible and high injection rates are used, usually 30 ml at 10–20 ml/s. For the higher rates, a central injection into the superior vena cava or right atrium is needed, making the procedure more invasive.

Large-vessel flow and cardiac shunts

Blood flow can be calculated as the product of mean velocity and cross-sectional area. The former can be derived from peak arrival times from time–density curves at multiple levels along the vessel, the latter by planimetry at any level [26]. Alternative approaches involve calculating the area under the curve after applying a gamma-variate fit to the time–attenuation curve for the cross-section of the vessel (see Chapter 4). This is then corrected for the attenuation increment produced by a known concentration of contrast medium. Garrett *et al.* [27] used this technique with the left-ventricular blood pool in dogs and showed a good correlation with cardiac output measurements by thermodilution. As might be expected, cardiac output measurements are equally valid when calculated using time–attenuation curves from the ascending aorta or pulmonary artery. Caution is advised, however, when using right-sided chambers for output measurements, as contrast mixing may be incomplete.

EBCT can provide exquisite detail of complex cardiac anatomy in congenital heart disease but, in the flow mode, has the added bonus of being able to quantify shunts. Adopting the same approach used by first-pass radionuclide ventriculography, pulmonary-to-systemic flow ratios can be calculated from the time–attenuation curve for any chamber or vessel distal to the shunt or from the lungs. The integrated areas of the two components of the bimodal curve are then used to determine shunt ratio (Figure 9.13) [28]. The method has been validated against values obtained from oxygen data using the Fick principle and holds for ratios between 1.3:1 and 2.5:1.

Myocardial perfusion

Rumberger *et al.* [29] were the first to use EBCT to measure myocardial perfusion *in vivo*. Using the Mullani–Gould equation [30] (see Chapter 4), regional myocardial perfusion was calculated from CT flow data and compared with perfusion measured using radiolabelled microspheres in dogs. Measurements were made before and after vasodilatation with intravenous adenosine. Calculated flow per unit mass ranged from 30–390 ml/min/100 g and correlated well with microsphere data at low flow rates. This was also the experience of Wolfkiel *et al.* [31] who found a near linear relationship up to 150 ml/min/100 g, but progressive underestimation above that. There are few studies in man, but results are similar [32,33]. Maximum flow reserve, as determined by EBCT in normal volunteers, was in the region of 2.7:1, whereas expected values from intravascular Doppler are closer to 5:1. The main causes for error fall into three categories: image and reconstruction artefacts; intramyocardial blood volume changes; and limitations of indicator dilution theory.

Image and reconstruction artefacts

As previously described, the geometry of an EBCT scanner causes non-linearity of attenuation number measurement across the field of view. This is most pronounced when adjacent regions differ substantially in attenuation coefficient. The X-ray beam is polychromatic and as it crosses areas of high attenuation, lower energy components are absorbed. The resulting beam has a higher proportion of high-energy photons (beam hardening) which are less efficiently detected. Photon scatter has a different aetiology but is also exaggerated by high attenuators in the beam. Reconstruction algorithms are designed to compensate for this effect, but when the attenuator is very dense, i.e. a contrast-enhanced ventricular blood pool, correction is inadequate. In the situation that pertains

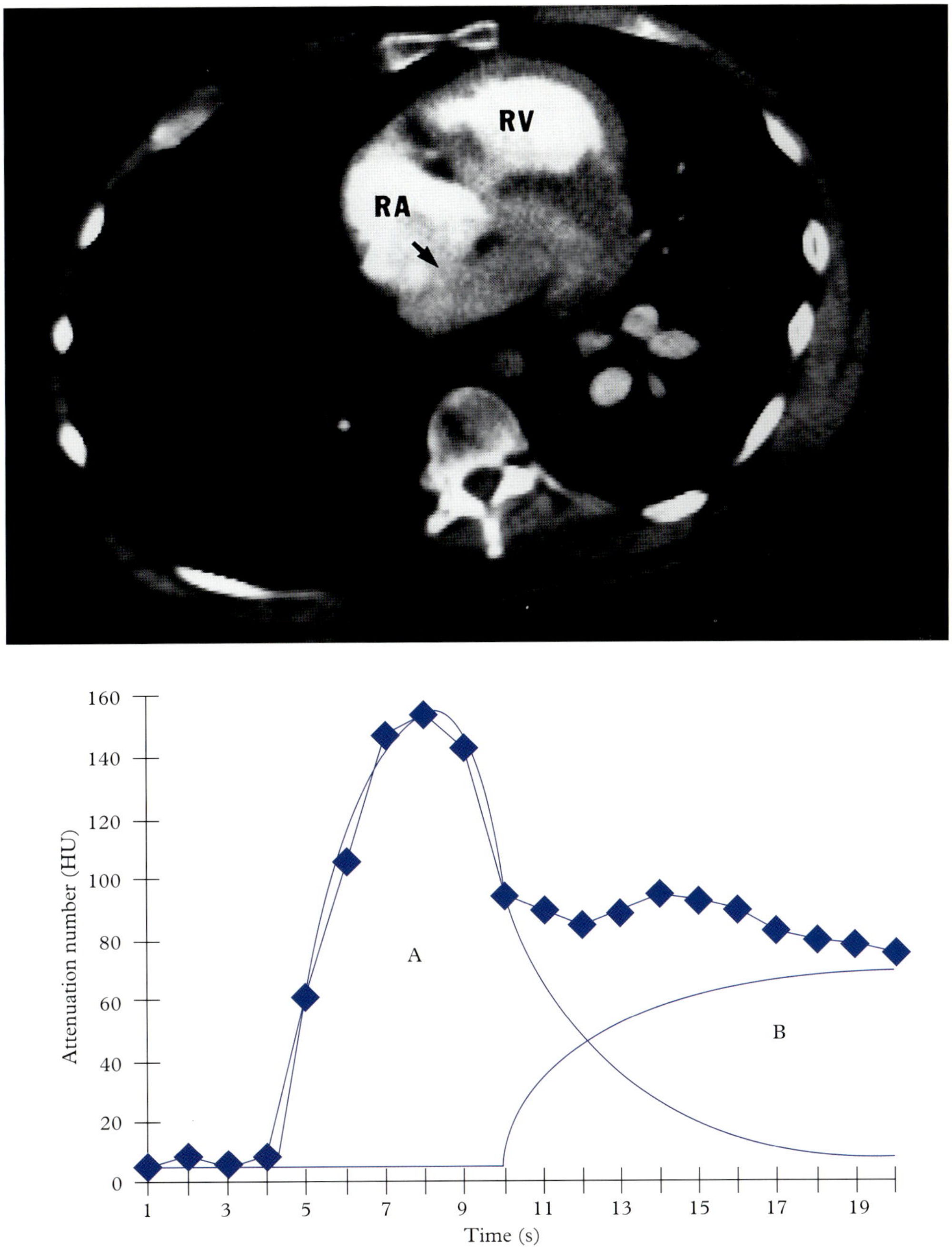

Figure 9.13
(a) Image from a contrast bolus-tracking sequence at the level of the interatrial septum. Right-sided cardiac chambers are enlarged (RA = right atrium, RV = right ventricle) and there is a large atrial septal defect (arrow). (b) For a ROI over the right atrium, the time–density curve during a contrast bolus is shown to be bimodal. Analysis with a gamma-variate fit gives two components, first pass (A) and early recirculation (B). From these the shunt ratio can be calculated. The Q_p:Q_s ratio = A/(A–B) (Q_p = pulmonary flow, Q_s = systemic flow).

when measuring myocardial perfusion with EBCT, the contrast-enhanced blood pool acts as a high attenuator in the centre of the ventricular muscle. This artificially reduces the enhancement seen in adjacent myocardium and is most marked where dose is lowest, i.e. anteriorly (Figure 9.14). As the contrast medium is washed out of the ventricle, beam hardening diminishes and the values for myocardial enhancement become more valid. The use of software corrections, a lower dose of contrast medium and minimizing scatter, by acquiring one slice instead of two, will all help to reduce this effect, but will not eliminate it.

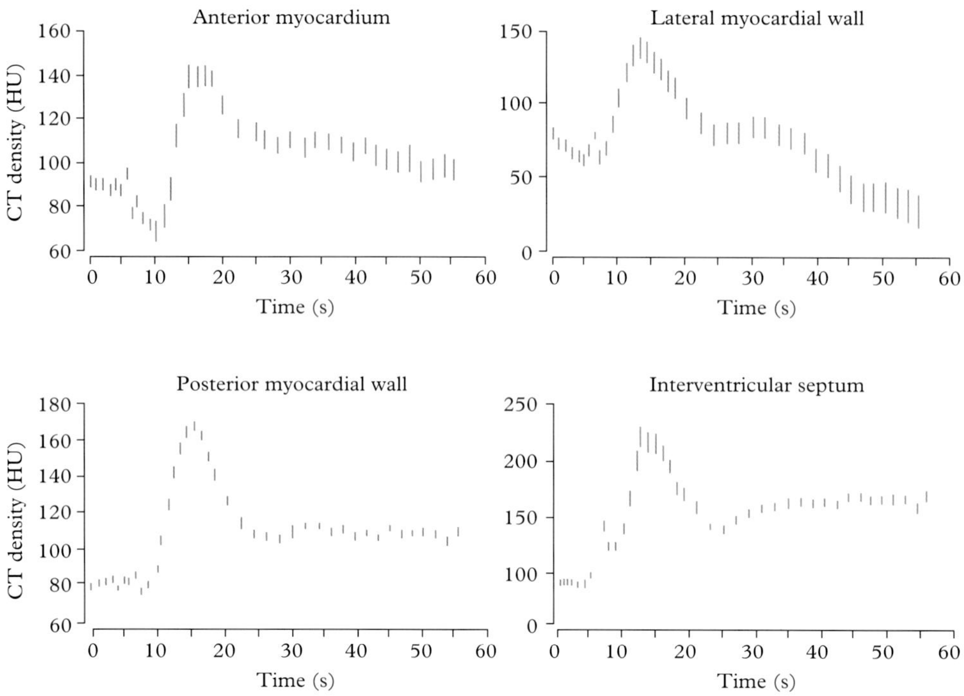

Figure 9.14
Simultaneous time–density curves for four ROIs within the left-ventricular myocardium of a dog during a bolus injection of contrast medium. Each datum point represents mean attenuation value ± standard deviation. Non-uniformity of the curves relates to asymmetric CT geometry and beam hardening; myocardial perfusion in all areas was normal. The dip in attenuation values below baseline for the anterior myocardium correlates with the presence of dense contrast medium in the left ventricle. (Reproduced with permission from J.A. Rumberger, A.J. Feiring and M.J. Lipton (1987) Use of ultrafast computed tomography to quantitate regional myocardial perfusion: a preliminary report. *Journal of the American College of Cardiology*, **9**, 59–72.)

Intramyocardial blood-volume changes

Several groups have explored the issue of intramyocardial blood volume. Myocardium is unusual when compared with other organs in that oxygen extraction from blood is maximal, even at rest. The only way to increase oxygen supply on exercise is to increase flow; increased extraction is not an option. As such, intramyocardial blood volume can vary enormously under different physiological conditions. At rest, most estimates suggest a blood volume of 4–7 ml/100 g of myocardium while at peak exercise this rises to 24 ml/g when maximally vasodilated. Failure to account for these changes will artificially underestimate myocardial perfusion in high-flow states and the effect will be proportional to flow rate. By applying a correction factor, for blood-volume changes, to Rumberger's original animal data, correlation with microsphere perfusion measurements improves over the whole physiological range [34]. Most investigators have used systole for myocardial-flow measurements, but this is also complicated by intramyocardial blood volume. There is a steep perfusion gradient across the myocardial wall in systole with almost zero flow in the subendocardium. Subendocardial blood volume is also reduced. Using only systolic flow data is therefore likely to underestimate perfusion.

Limitations of indicator dye-dilution theory

Several assumptions must hold if the Mullani–Gould equation is to be valid in the setting of myocardial perfusion. Two are particularly significant. The indicator must not disturb the haemodynamics of the circulation it is being used to measure and there must be no loss of indicator from the region of interest before peak opacification.

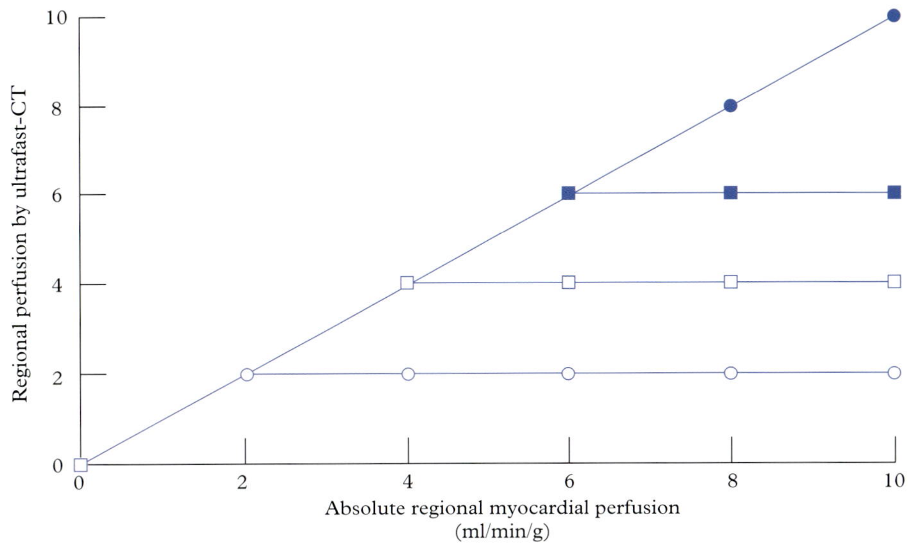

Figure 9.15
Graphical representation of the peak value of regional perfusion that can be estimated by EBCT for various injection sites. As the site of injection is brought closer to the systemic circulation, the bolus becomes more compact allowing measurement of higher levels of peak perfusion. For peak myocardial perfusion, levels of 5–6 ml/min/g, only injection in the aortic root is adequate. ○ = Femoral vein injection; □ = IVC injection; ■ = pulmonary artery injection; ● = aortic root injection. (Reproduced with permission from J.A. Rumberger, W. Stanford and M.L. Marcus (1987) Quantitation of regional myocardial perfusion by ultrafast CT: promises and pitfalls. *American Journal of Cardiac Imaging*, **1**, 336–344.

Intravascular contrast media are well known for the flushing, tachycardia and hypotension they produce. These effects can be minimized by using non-ionic media, but are not eliminated. While the contribution of these effects to the underestimate of perfusion are unknown, it is presumed to be small for low doses. Of greater importance is the assumption that the contrast bolus entering the coronary arteries is complete before contrast escapes into the coronary sinus, i.e. input function is shorter than transit time. This may be true at rest but as perfusion increases, increased blood velocity more than compensates for increased myocardial blood volume and transit time falls. It becomes impossible to provide a short enough input bolus from the intravenous route. The injection profile of contrast media given via a power injector approximates to a square wave. After passing through the pulmonary circulation, however, it becomes splayed, the degree of splaying being directly related to the site of injection. The more peripheral the injection site within the venous system, the more it will be splayed and the lower the peak myocardial perfusion that can be measured (Figure 9.15). Perfusion measurements have been made with direct injection of contrast medium into the aortic root. This provides the best input function, eliminates contrast within the ventricle and does give reliable results, but it is at the expense of a more invasive procedure. Alternative approaches to data analysis, possibly using peak gradients of enhancement rather than peak enhancement, may be more fruitful.

SUMMARY

The Imatron C100, and more recently the Evolution XP, are the first representatives of fifth-generation CT. By combining the high spatial resolution inherent in CT with greatly improved temporal resolution, they are ideally suited to cardiac imaging. An EBCT system can operate in three modes:

(i) volume mode, (ii) cine mode and (iii) flow mode. The combination of these three modes can be used to provide information about cardiac structure, function and perfusion in a way that no other modality can. Cine EBCT is used for estimating cardiac chamber volumes, myocardial mass and assessing regional wall motion. The methods are well validated and are the most accurate currently available. Studies in the flow mode are used to calculate cardiac output, large-vessel flow and tissue perfusion. While myocardial perfusion can be measured with reasonable accuracy at rest, problems with scanner geometry and contrast delivery lead to underestimates of perfusion in the vasodilated state. Time will tell whether these problems can be solved but it seems more likely that alternative technologies will be developed before EBCT can provide the answers.

REFERENCES

1. Garcia, E.V. (1991) Physics and instrumentation of radionuclide imaging. In: *Cardiac Imaging — A Companion to Braunwald's Heart Disease* (eds M.L. Marcus, D.J. Skorton, H.R. Schelbert *et al.*), pp. 977–1005. Philadelphia: W.B. Saunders.
2. Boyd, D.P. and Lipton, M.J. (1983) Cardiac computed tomography. *Proceedings of the IEEE*, **71**, 305–320.
3. McCollough, C.H. and Morin, R.L. (1994) The technical design and performance of ultrafast computed tomography. *Radiology Clinics of North America*, **32**, 521–526.
4. Rumberger, J.A. (1992) Ultrafast computed tomography scanning modes, scanning planes and practical aspects of contrast administration. In: *Ultrafast Computed Tomography in Cardiac Imaging* (eds W. Stanford and J.A. Rumberger), p. 17. Mount Kisko, NY: Futura.
5. Diethelm, L., Simonson, J.S., Dery, R. *et al.* (1989) Determination of left ventricular mass with ultrafast CT and 2-dimensional echocardiography. *Radiology*, **171**, 213–217.
6. Reiter, S.J., Rumberger, J.A., Feiring, A.J. *et al.* (1986) Precision of right and left ventricular stroke volume measurements by rapid acquisition cine computed tomography. *Circulation*, **74**, 890–900.
7. Feiring, A., Rumberger, J.A., Reiter, S.J. *et al.* (1985) Determination of left ventricular mass in dogs with rapid acquisition cardiac computed tomographic scanning. *Circulation*, **6**, 1355–1361.
8. Hoffman, K.R., Chen, S-Y., Kormano, M. *et al.* (1993) Segmentation and display of hepatic vessels and metastases. *Proceedings of SPIE*, 1898, 262–270.
9. Furst, M.A. and Caines, P.E. (1986) Edge detection with image enhancement via dynamic programming. *Computer Vision, Graphics and Image Processing*, **33**, 263–279.
10. Feigle, S.R., Thedens, D.R., Ehrhardt, J.C. *et al.* (1991) Automated identification of left ventricular borders from spin-echo magnetic images. *Investigative Radiology*, **26**, 295–303.
11. Feng, J., Lin, W.C. and Chen, C-T. (1990) Automatic left ventricular boundary detection in digital 2-dimensional echocardiography using fuzzy reasoning techniques. *Proceedings of SPIE Conference on Biomedical Image Processing*, 1245, 19–105.
12. Chu, C.H., Delp, E.J. and Buda, A.J. (1988) Detecting left ventricular endocardial and epicardial boundaries by digital 2-dimensional echocardiography. *IEEE Transactions on Medical Imaging*, **7**, 81–90.

13. Hayball, M.P., Coulden, R.A., Lee, E. and Lomas, D.J. (1996) A semi-automated tool for the measurement of left ventricular function from magnetic resonance. *Proceedings of Computer Aided Radiology*, 121–124.
14. Graves, M.J., Powell, S.A. and Heron, C.W. (1994) Evaluation of ventricular volume measurements with breath-hold cine MRI and stereological analysis. *Proceedings of the Society of Magnetic Resonance*, **1**, 205.
15. Ringertz, H.G., Rodgers, B., Lipton, M.J. *et al.* (1985) Assessment of human right ventricular cast volume by CT and angiocardiography. *Investigative Radiology*, **20**, 29–32.
16. Lipton, M.J., Hayashi, T.T., Boyd, D. *et al.* (1987) Measurement of left ventricular cast volume by computed tomography. *Radiology*, **127**, 419–424.
17. Reiter, S.J., Rumberger, J.A., Feiring, A.J. *et al.* (1986) Precision of right and left ventricular stroke volume measurements by rapid acquisition cine computed tomography. *Circulation*, **74**, 890–900.
18. Reiter, S.J., Rumberger, J.A., Stanford, W. *et al.* (1987) Quantitative determination of aortic regurgitant volumes by cine computed tomography. *Circulation*, **76**, 728–735.
19. Lipton, M.J. and Rumberger, A.J. (1991) The assessment of left ventricular systolic and diastolic function by ultrafast computed tomography. *American Journal of Cardiac Imaging*, **5**, 318–327.
20. Rumberger, J.A., Weiss, R.M., Feiring, A.J. *et al.* (1989) Patterns of regional diastolic function in the normal human left ventricle: an ultrafast computed tomographic study. *Journal of the American College of Cardiology*, **14**, 119–126.
21. Marzullo, P., L'Abbate, A. and Marcus, M.L. (1991) Patterns of global and regional systolic and diastolic function in the normal right ventricle assessed by ultrafast computed tomography. *Journal of the American College of Cardiology*, **17**, 1318–1325.
22. Roig, E., Georgiou, D., Chomka, E.V. *et al.* (1991) Reproducibility of left ventricular myocardial volume and mass measurements by ultrafast computed tomography. *Journal of the American College of Cardiology*, **18**, 990–996.
23. Hajduczok, Z., Weiss, R.M., Stanford, W. *et al.* (1990) Determination of right ventricular mass in dogs with ultrafast cardiac computed tomography. *Circulation*, **82**, 202–212.
24. Lessick, J., Sideman, S., Azhari, H. *et al.* (1991) Regional three-dimensional geometry and function of left ventricles with fibrous aneurysms — a cine computed tomography study. *Circulation*, **84**, 1072–1086.
25. Kocke, F.J. (1987) Measurements of coronary flow reserve: defining pathophysiology vs. making decisions about patient care. *Circulation*, **76**, 1183–1189.
26. Ringertz, H., Jashke, W., Sievers, R.E. *et al.* (1987) Relative carotid blood flow measurements in dogs by high-speed CT. *Investigative Radiology*, **22**, 960–964.
27. Garrett, J.S., Lanzer, P., Jaschke, W. *et al.* (1985) Measurement of cardiac output by cine computed tomography. *American Journal of Cardiology*, **56**, 657–661.
28. Eldridge, J.W. (1991) Comprehensive evaluation of congenital heart disease using ultrafast computed tomography. In: *Cardiac Imaging — A Companion to Braunwald's Heart Disease* (eds M.L. Marcus, D.J. Skorton, H.R. Schelbert *et al.*), pp. 715–731. Philadelphia: WB Saunders.
29. Rumberger, J.A., Feiring, A.J. and Lipton, M.J. (1987) Use of ultrafast computed tomography to quantitate regional myocardial perfusion: a preliminary report. *Journal of the American College of Cardiology*, **9**, 59–72.

30. Mullani, N., Goldstein, R.A., Gould, K.L. *et al.* (1983) Myocardial perfusion maesurements with rubidium-82. I. Measurements of extraction fraction and flow with external detectors. *Journal of Nuclear Medicine*, **24**, 898–911.
31. Wolfkiel, C.J., Ferguson, J.L., Chomka, E.V. *et al.* (1987) Measurement of myocardial blood flow by ultrafast computed tomography. *Circulation*, **76**, 1262–1273.
32. Rumberger, J.A., Stanford, W. and Marcus, M.L. (1987) Quantitation of regional myocardial perfusion by ultrafast CT: Promises and pitfalls. *American Journal of Cardiac Imaging*, **1**, 336–344.
33. Ludman, P.F., Coats, A.J.S., Burger, P. *et al.* (1993) Validation of measurement of regional myocardial perfusion in humans by ultrafast X-ray computed tomography. *American Journal of Cardiac Imaging*, **7**, 267–279.
34. Rumberger, J.A., Bell, M.R., Feiring, A.J. *et al.* (1991) Measurement of myocardial perfusion using ultrafast computed tomography. In: *Cardiac Imaging — A Companion to Braunwald's Heart Disease* (eds M.L. Marcus, D.J. Skorton, H.R. Schelbert *et al.*) pp. 688–702. Philadelphia: W.B. Saunders.

Chapter 10

CT PERMEABILITY IMAGING: BLOOD–BRAIN BARRIER IMAGING

K. Miles and P. Dawson

INTRODUCTION

The permeability of blood vessels is an index of considerable physiological and pathophysiological significance but one not readily measured. As will be shown in this chapter, it may be measured/imaged using dynamic contrast enhanced computed tomography (CT).

Unlike perfusion imaging which uses a first-pass technique during which the contrast medium remains predominantly intravascular, permeability studies use a longer protocol to allow the contrast medium to leak out of the vascular system into the extravascular space. Qualitative analysis of time–density curves has been used to assess the permeability of brain tumours [1] but absolute quantification of capillary permeability is achievable with appropriate analysis of the temporal changes in tissue and vascular concentrations of iodine, as determined by attenuation measurements (see Chapter 4). Depending upon the analysis used, it is possible to measure the rate constants for passage both from intravascular to extravascular (K_1) and also from extravascular to intravascular (K_2) [2,3]. However, to determine K_1 only, a simpler, shorter protocol can be used [4]. Generally, CT techniques for measuring permeability have only been used to study blood–brain barrier (BBB) permeability, but permeability measurements in other tissues are potentially of value also.

SOME THEORETICAL CONSIDERATIONS

An indication of the possible theoretical approach to the study of capillary permeability may be seen from the following. Let the rate constants for mass transfer of contrast agent from blood to interstitium and back again be, respectively, K_1 and K_2. Let $b(t)$ and $C_{is}(t)$ be the concentrations of contrast agent at any time, t, in blood and interstitium, respectively. Let $Q_b(t)$ and $Q_{is}(t)$ be the masses of contrast agent in the two spaces.

Then we may write

$$\frac{dQ_{is}(t)}{dt} = K_1 b(t) - K_2 C_{is}(t) \tag{1}$$

$$\frac{dQ_b(t)}{dt} = K_1 b(t) + K_2 C_{is}(t) \tag{2}$$

If, for the moment, we consider the early phase when K_1 dominates, Equation (1) yields

$$\frac{dQ_{is}(t)}{dt} = K_1 b(t)$$

Dividing by V, the volume of the region of interest (ROI)

$$\frac{1}{V}\frac{dQ_{is}(t)}{dt} = \frac{K_1}{V}\cdot b(t)$$

This is the effective contribution of interstitial contrast to the total concentration in the ROI.

After a time period we have

$$\text{contribution to concentration} = \frac{K_1}{V}\int_0^t b(t)dt$$

Let ϕ_b be the proportionate vascular volume in the ROI, in which case the effective contribution of contrast in blood will be $\phi_b b(t)$. The total effective concentration at any time, t, will therefore be

$$c(t) = \frac{K_1}{V}\int_0^t b(t)dt + \phi_b b(t) \tag{3}$$

K_1/V is the mass transfer contrast per unit volume. Its units are ml/min/ml. K_1/V is, in fact, the PS-product per unit volume of the physiologist. This equation may be used to model enhancement curves such as those seen in breast lesions. Such enhancement curves clearly reflect a number of important tumour tissue properties including capillary permeability.

To proceed further we follow the mathematical approach outlined in Chapters 3 and 8 by dividing (3) throughout by $b(t)$ to obtain

$$\frac{c(t)}{b(t)} = \frac{K_1}{V}\frac{\int_0^t b(t)dt}{b(t)} + \phi_b$$

Comparing this with Equation (7) of Chapter 3 (page 39) we see that, entirely reasonably,

$$\phi_{is}C_{is}(t) = \frac{K_1}{V}\int_0^t b(t)dt$$

Now, a plot of

$$\frac{c(t)}{b(t)} \text{ versus } \frac{\int_0^t b(t)\mathrm{d}t}{b(t)}$$

will, after an initial (variable) period during which tracer/contrast-free blood is replaced by tracer-containing blood, yield, initially, a straight line of slope K_1/V and (extrapolated) intercept ϕ_b on the ordinate (see Chapter 3, Figure 3.17, page 41).

If such a plot is carried out using data from enhancing normal brain the result is, of course, a line of gradient close to zero

$$\frac{c(t)}{b(t)} = \phi_\mathrm{b}$$

The line has a close to zero gradient since $K_1/V \approx 0$ for the intact BBB.

Effect of K_2

In the early phase following contrast-agent administration, contrast transfer is from blood to interstitium. Later, as blood levels fall, contrast returns from the interstitium to blood at a rate determined by K_2. In general, $K_1 \neq K_2$. In this case, the solution of Equations (1) and (2) becomes a little more difficult, but the following solution may be obtained.

$$\frac{c(t)}{b(t)} = \frac{\frac{K_1}{V}\left[\mathrm{e}^{-K_2 t}\int_0^t \mathrm{e}^{-K_2 t} b(t)\mathrm{d}t\right]}{b(t)} + \phi_\mathrm{b}$$

A plot of $c(t)/b(t)$ versus t now deviates from the initial linearity and becomes asymptotic to $\phi_\mathrm{b} + \phi_\mathrm{is}/(1 - \mathrm{Hct})$ as indicated in Chapter 3.

BLOOD–BRAIN BARRIER PERMEABILITY

Technique

As with perfusion imaging, protocols use a single-location dynamic sequence but with a longer total imaging time and longer delays between individual data acquisitions. As no rapid imaging is entailed, it is not necessary to use modern spiral CT equipment for this technique which can theoretically be performed on almost any CT machine. However, with the longer interscan delay, the use of spiral systems would allow repeated volume acquisitions and calculation of three-dimensional permeability datasets rather than the more common single-slice technique. Off course, the higher radiation burden would have to be taken into consideration.

For measurement of K_1 and K_2 a baseline image followed by serial imaging, for 30–40 min after intravenous contrast medium administration, is required. Calculation of BBB permeability is achieved using values of blood and brain attenuation from each image in the sequence and non-linear regression analysis [2,3]. The simpler method which determines K_1 alone requires only 5 min of imaging with permeability determined from Patlak plots (see Chapter 4). Within the first few minutes, very little contrast medium has left the vascular space and therefore the amount returning from the extravascular system can be considered negligible. As both protocols are over a much longer time than those for perfusion imaging, movement between images is more likely to occur than with perfusion imaging. Therefore, careful immobilization and instruction of the patient is essential for a high-quality study. For either method, pixel-by-pixel analysis can be used to create functional images mapping BBB permeability.

Both methods require measurement of vascular concentrations of contrast medium for which the most reliable method is to determine the attenuation of serial arterial blood samples taken from the patient. However, this makes the examination somewhat invasive and thus less generally applicable. Determination of arterial concentration from CT images of the brain is also difficult because the cerebral vessels are small and prone to partial volume effects leading to underestimation of the vascular concentration. This effect can be minimized by using an edge detection algorithm for determination of a vascular ROI (see below).

Imaging sequence

As with perfusion imaging, the choice of imaging sequence is a balance between temporal sampling rate and radiation burden. A baseline image containing the area of interest is performed and the contrast medium injection started simultaneously. The rate and volume of injection are not critical but the author uses 50 ml of Iopamidol 300 mg/ml over 15 s. (To some extent, the value of permeability measured will be dependent upon the molecular weight of the contrast medium.) For a K_1-only study, the following sequence is suitable: 0, 20, 40, 60, 80, 100, 120, 150, 180, 240, 300 s. The 20 s image is useful for vessel identification (see below). The acquisitions are more frequent within the first 2 min, which is the period of minimal return of contrast medium from the extravascular system. For structures with very low permeability, such as normal brain, the period over which return from the extravascular space remains insignificant will be longer whilst the Patlak plots (see below) are improved by the additional later time points. Compressing the image matrix to 256×256 followed by spatial smoothing (the author uses four iterations of a standard nine-point smooth) will reduce the effects of photon noise in the subsequent analysis.

Vessel identification

The edge detection method used by the author initially involves generation of two parametric images: peak enhancement and time to peak enhancement. The vessels appear as areas of greatest and earliest enhancement. A ROI is drawn around the most enhancing vessel. The edge detection algorithm then identifies the most enhancing pixel within the ROI and includes all adjacent pixels with a peak enhancement value within 10% and a time to peak enhancement within 3 s of the most enhancing pixel. Typically, the final ROI will contain approximately 10 pixels (256×256 matrix).

Region of interest analysis

A ROI is drawn around the brain area to be evaluated and serial measurements of attenuation are made. These are used along with similar data from the vascular

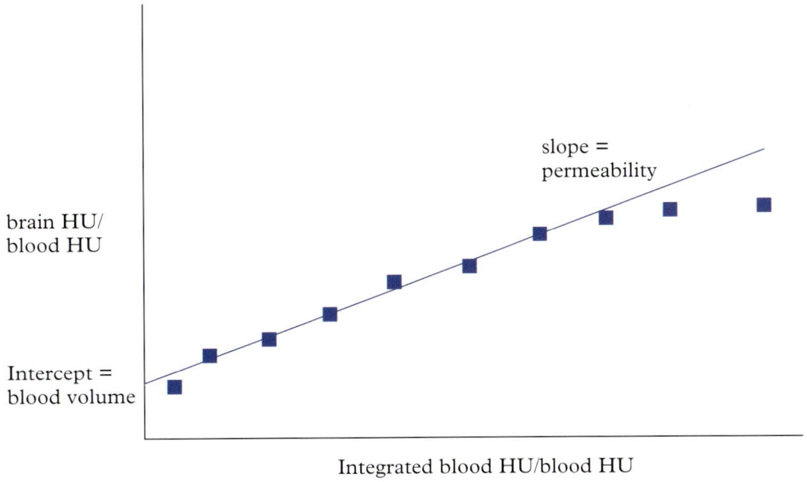

Figure 10.1
Patlak plot of CT data from a brain tumour.

ROI to create the Patlak plot, displaying brain attenuation divided by blood attenuation on the *y*-axis and the time-integrated blood attenuation divided by blood attenuation on the *x*-axis. The operator inspects the plot to identify the points that form the straight-line portion of the plot (Figure 10.1). These points are then used to generate a straight line using a standard least-squares fit. The gradient of the line yields the permeability, the intercept with the *y*-axis the relative blood volume of the brain region studied.

Functional images of blood–brain barrier permeability

With a suitable computer program, the above analysis can be performed pixel by pixel to create a BBB permeability image. It is clearly impractical to determine the extent of the linear fit for individual pixels. Therefore, a ROI analysis is performed as above to determine the limits of the linear fit which is then applied uniformly to all the individual pixels. The brain ROI chosen for this purpose should be from an area, such as a brain tumour, in which the permeability is anticipated to be high. This is because the Patlak plots from areas of highest permeability will fall away from a straight-line sooner due to the more rapid increase in the amount of extravascular contrast medium. If the subsequent permeability image shows that the chosen ROI was not the most permeable region, then the functional image can be used to define a new ROI and the analysis repeated.

Two functional images are obtained: permeability and blood volume. By mathematically separating extravascular and intravascular components of contrast enhancement, the functional images reveal information that cannot be assessed intuitively by visual inspection of conventional enhanced CT images. In the context of assessing BBB permeability, the intravascular information effectively creates noise which is removed by the Patlak analysis. In another clinical setting, such as cerebrovascular disease, the blood-volume images could contain diagnostic information in their own right. The final BBB permeability images (Figure 10.2) demonstrate the choroid plexuses as areas of high permeability as these are outside the BBB. Normal brain exhibits very low permeability whereas tumours are seen as areas of high permeability, due to the associated disruption of the BBB.

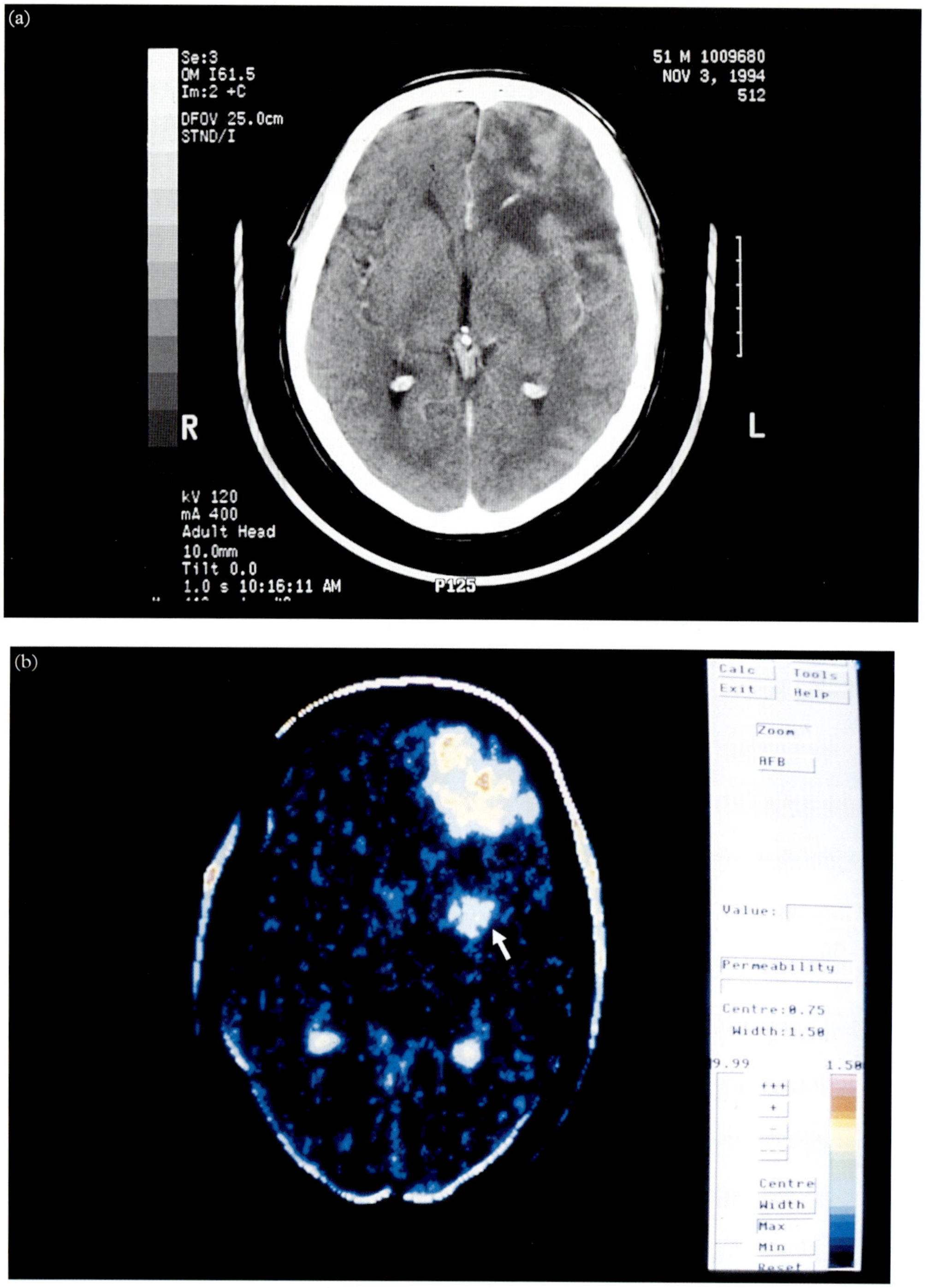

Figure 10.2
(a) Conventional enhanced CT, (b) BBB-permeability image (c) blood-volume image and in a patient with a recurrent left frontal glioma. Note the second tumour nidus (arrow) seen on the BBB-permeability image but not on the conventional CT. This was confirmed by gadolinium-enhanced MR. The choroid plexuses are seen posteriorly.

APPLICATIONS OF BLOOD–BRAIN BARRIER IMAGING

To date, studies using CT permeability measurements have been restricted to the study of brain tumours. However, the technique has potential value in assessing the severity or activity of other brain conditions such as cerebral ischaemia or demyelinating diseases.

Figure 10.2
(continued)

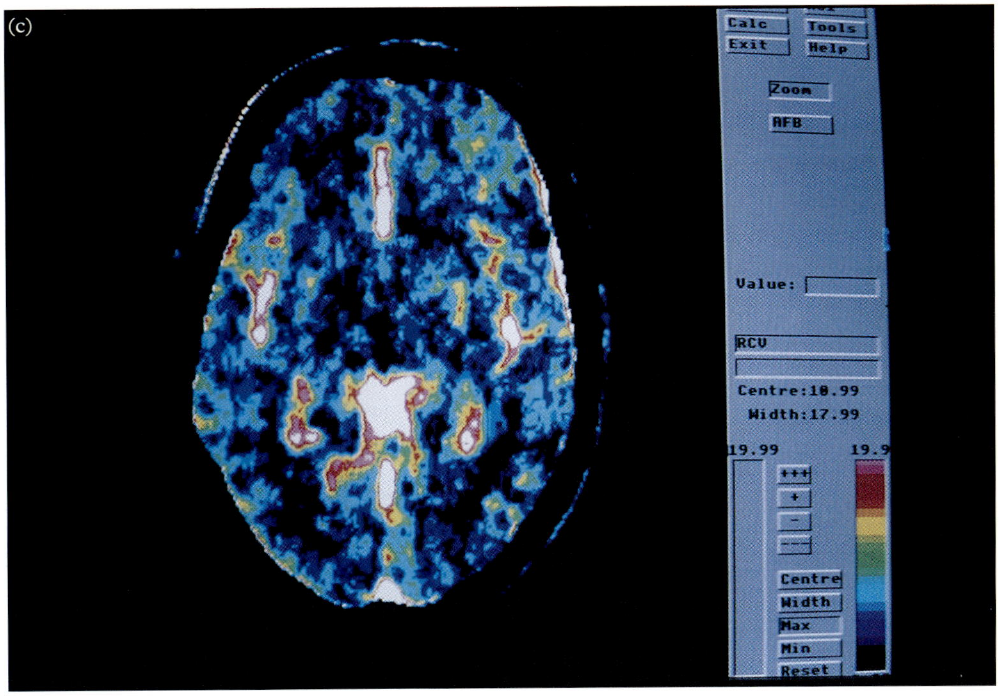

Table 10.1
Blood–brain barrier permeability measurements in brain tumours

Study		Tumour K_1 (μl/min/ml)	Normal brain (μl/min/ml)
Groothius *et al.* [2]	Glioma	2.0–33.9	1.7–5.4
Yeung *et al.* [3]	Glioma and metastases	27.3 ± 6.0	1.9 ± 1.5
Yeung *et al.* [5]	Glioma	0.0–25.3	0–1.0
	Meningioma	57.5–462	—
Miles *et al.* [4]	Glioma	14.0–46.0	0–3.0

The interest in brain tumours has resulted because of the importance of the extent of brain-barrier disruption, caused by the tumour, in determining the local delivery of chemotherapeutic agents. All studies have shown significantly increased permeability within a variety of brain tumours as compared with normal brain in humans (Table 10.1). The results of the different studies are generally in agreement. Comparison between CT and positron emission tomography (PET) measurements of BBB permeability cannot be made due to the difference in size of tracer molecule.

The effect of drugs on BBB permeability is also an important issue. Yeung *et al.* [5] used CT permeability imaging to demonstrate that steroid medication given to reduce cerebral oedema in patients with tumours also reduces the

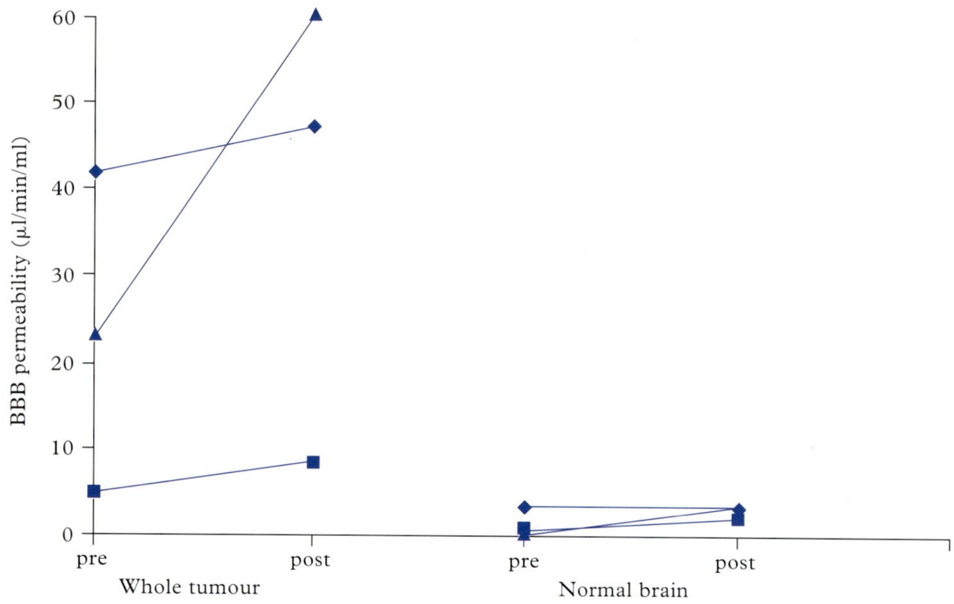

Figure 10.3
The effects of the bradykinin analogue RMP-7 on the permeability of cerebral gliomas and normal brain as determined by CT permeability measurements. The permeability of gliomas is increased whereas normal brain is unaffected. ▲ = Patient 1; ◆ = patient 2; ■ = patient 3.

permeability of the tumour. Whereas this may be the mechanism of the anti-oedema effect of steroids, it may also reduce delivery of chemotherapeutic agents to the brain tumour. Pharmacological modification of the BBB to increase permeability, and therefore chemotherapeutic drug delivery, has been proposed. Figure 10.3 demonstrates the increase in BBB permeability induced by the bradykinin analogue RMP-7 (Alkermes Europe) in a series of patients undergoing carboplatin chemotherapy for cerebral glioma. Significant increases in permeability occur but with no measurable effect on normal brain regions.

Functional images of BBB permeability have demonstrated heterogeneity of permeability within tumours. It also dramatically improves the delineation of tumour when compared to conventional contrast enhanced CT and may allow visualization of lesions not apparent on unprocessed CT images (Figure 10.2). This has implications for radiotherapy planning so that the full extent of the tumour is included within the radiotherapy field. The technique is also of potential use in planning stereotaxic biopsy of brain lesions allowing biopsy of the most permeable area of the tumour.

SUMMARY

The use of CT to measure capillary permeability has many advantages. Only conventional equipment and contrast media are necessary and so the technique is much more readily available than PET, the only other method for absolute measurement of BBB permeability. The technique is easily incorporated into current CT imaging protocols allowing an anatomical and permeability assessment in one investigation. The high spatial resolution allows accurate placement of ROIs for study and provides functional images with a resolution superior to PET images. The technique has not been fully evaluated but early indications are that it is of potential value in neuro-imaging. It could also have applications in imaging other body regions.

REFERENCES

1. Terada, T., Nishiguchi, T., Hyoutani, G. *et al.* (1989) A study on the vascular permeability of brain tumors using dynamic CT (in Japanese). *No Shinkei Geka*, **17**, 841–848.
2. Groothius, D.R., Vriesendorp, F.J., Kupfer, B. *et al.* (1991) Quantitative measurements of capillary transport in human brain tumours by computed tomography. *Annals of Neurology*, **30**, 581–588.
3. Yeung, W.T.I., Lee, T-Y., Del Maestro, R.F. *et al.* (1992) *In vivo* CT measurement of blood–brain transfer constant of iopamidol in human brain tumors. *Journal of Neuro-oncology*, **14**, 177–187.
4. Ford, J.M., Miles, K.A, Hayball, M.P, Bearcroft, P.W, Bleehen, N.M. and Osborn, C.S. (1996) A simplified technique for measurement of blood-brain barrier permeability using CT: preliminary results and the effect of RMP-7. Qualitative Imaging in Oncology, Proceedings of the 19th LH Grey Conference. Br J Radiol, 1–5.
5. Yeung, W.T.I., Lee, T-Y., Del Maestro, R.F. *et al.* (1994) Effect of steroids on iopamidol blood–brain transfer constant and plasma volume in brain tumours measured with X-ray computed tomography. *Journal of Neuro-oncology*, **18**, 53–60.

INDEX